DEDICATION

I would first like to applaud every reader of this book-let for considering an alternative lifestyle towards better health.

I would personally thank Phil Allen who originally wrote this booklet, for his inspiration, research and focus when Handy Pantry Distributors was in its infancy.

And finally, Ann Wigmore and Victoras Kulvinskas for their inspiration and direction back in the '70s before anyone knew anything.

This updated version of *Sprouting for Health in the New Millennium* is offered by Living Whole Foods with the new title ***Wheatgrass, Sprouts, Microgreens, and the Living Food Diet*** to acknowledge the increasing aware-ness of the importance of each. More people are opting for a healthy diet, so all the information needed to grow grasses and greens, as well as to sprout, is in one booklet.

We would like to acknowledge the work of Dr. Ann Wig-more in developing and promoting these foods as a major and important part of her vegan dietary system, which also included fermented and wild foods, sea vegetables, juices, raw soups, and smoothies, all of which make eating as enjoyable as it is healthy.

All the folks at **Living Whole Foods, Inc.** (2010) wish you

GOOD HEALTH AND HAPPY GROWING!

WHEATGRASS, SPROUTS, MICROGREENS,

AND THE LIVING FOOD DIET

by Living Whole Foods, Inc.

WELCOME
TO THE NEW MILLENNIUM

In the advent of the last decade, *Sprouting For Health in the 90s* had managed to survive 10 years of scrutiny and changes. Throughout the following pages, you will find not only helpful methods of detoxifying the chemical soup that many of us live in, but also new sprouting beans and grains available, tray sprouting methods (wheatgrass, sunflower, etc.), how to grow and use sprouts, recipes and more.

Wheatgrass, Sprouts, Microgreens, and the Living Food Diet is our latest update of this time tested classic work.

We know that many of our readers share their copy with family and friends. Therefore, we consider it our obligation to offer up-to-date information on the subject of sprouting and growing. Look for our sprouting education centers in your local retail stores.

We would personally like to thank all of our readers for their continued support throughout the years with your questions, comments, compliments and suggestions. E-Mail us if you'd like to at support@wheatgrasskits.com, or visit us on the web at www.wheatgrasskits.com. We would truly like to hear from you!

STAFF AND MANAGEMENT, LIVING WHOLE FOODS, INC.

Wheatgrass, Sprouts, Microgreens, and the Living Food Diet is solely for informational and educational purposes. No statement or part of this booklet is intended to diagnose or prescribe or take the place of a qualified physician. If you suspect chemical allergy, consult a health professional qualified in treating ecological illness.

Compiled by KK Fowlkes and Chuck Juhn
Published by Living Whole Foods, Inc.
1041 North 450 West, Springville Utah 84663
(801) 491-8700

TABLE OF CONTENTS

INTRODUCTION
HEALTH IN THE NEW MILLENNIUM

This book is about miracles. Tiny ones that we sometimes overlook. Like that little cut on our finger. How miraculous. It heals itself! Sometimes though, due to our carelessness, it becomes infected, and begins to give us pain. Pain is our body's signal to us that it needs help. With a cut finger the course of action is obvious. Clean it and disinfect it. But what about tiny, invisible "cuts" that we can't see, which are happening inside our bodies all the time? What do we do about subtle messages of pain coming from them? Too many of us reach for the nearest chemical "pain-reliever," when we could be doing something more—and better. Poor health stalks our nation.

A FACT OF HEALTH

A body that is toxic is like a cut with dirt in it. It is contaminated and may not heal properly. It needs to be cleaned and given the nutrients it needs to disinfect, detoxify, rebuild, and heal itself. Many of us have already recognized this fact of life and have altered our lifestyles to avoid as many chemicals as possible. Some of us have also recognized this fact of health and we are being more careful about our nutrition. There is a food source in nature full of concentrated nutrients that can help our body detoxify and rebuild our immune system. It is **chlorophyll**.

A FACT OF LIFE

Our bodies are being damaged inside, invisibly and mercilessly, by toxic, chemical reactions. Toxic chemical additives and hazardous wastes in our air, water, and food supplies will continue to degrade our living and working environments. These toxins are contained in everything we eat, drink, and breathe. Thankfully, much of the internal damage they do heals automatically, like that cut on our finger. However, when our body is not adequately nourished it can't neutralize and expel these poisons fast enough. They build up in our body; and so does the invisible damage they do. Toxic buildup can severely damage our immune system.

THE WHEATGRASS STORY

Growing wheatgrass, buckwheat and sunflower sprouts as well as juicing them stems back to the 1970s to Ann Wigmore and Victoras Kulvinskas. The Boston Institute of Health advocated these methods long before it became a national fad. Ann Wigmore was a hero in the natural heath movement and left a legacy of books such as *The Wheatgrass Book*, *The Sprouting Book*, *The Blending Book* and others. Ann was a researcher and a humanitarian and even went to India to spread her message.

This is the new era of juicing for health and almost everyone has heard of wheatgrass by now. The following information offers a much requested statistical analysis on the subject. The structural breakdown of Wheatgrass is so concentrated that one ounce of Wheatgrass has the same nutritional value as 2.5 pounds of green garden vegetables.

There are many other benefits to be found in wheatgrass besides vitamins, minerals, and amino acids, these include:

chlorophyll, known for its ability to nourish the blood and detoxify poisons, enzymes that help the digestion and metabolization of nutrients and abscissic acid which is known for its anti-tumor activity.

Growing wheatgrass need not be more complicated than these simple instructions, however look at our website at www.wheatgrasskits.com for updated information on wheatgrass cultivation.

It also contains more information about using wheatgrass, greens, and sprouts, especially in our archive of newsletters and testimonials. Remember, growing and sprouting is fun and easy when you know how!

WHEATGRASS NUTRITIONAL INFORMATION

One ounce of wheatgrass juice contains the following:

NUTRIENTS		VITAMINS	
protein	6,480 mg	A	14.175 IU
crude fiber	4,860 mg	K	2.268 mcg
calories	81	C	89.1 mg
chlorophyll	153.9 mg	thiamine	81 mcg
carbohydrates	10.53 mg	choline	8.1 mg
		riboflavin	575.1 mcg
AMINO ACIDS		pyroxidine	364.5 mcg
lysine	234.9 mg	vitamin B-12	8.1 mcg
		niacin	2,130.3 mcg
histidine	129.6 mg	pantothenic	680.4 mcg
arginine	315.9 mg	biotin	32.4 mcg
		folic acid	307.8 mcg
threonine	299.7 mg	**MINERALS**	
lutamic acid	688.5 mg	calcium	145.8 mg
proline	267.3 mg	phosphorus	145.8 mg
glycine	332.1 mg	potassium	907.2 mg
alanine	388.8 mg	magnesium	29.16 mg
valine	356.4 mg	iron	16.2 mg
isoleucin	251.1 mg	manganese	2.835 mg
leucine	461.7 mg	selenium	28.35 mcg
tyrosine	145.8 mg	sodium	8.1 mg
pheny lalinine	307.8 mg	zinc	141.75 mcg
methionnine	121.5 mg	iodine	56.7 mcg
cystine	64.8 mg	copper	0.162 mg
tryptophan	32.4 mg	cobalt	14.175 mcg
amide	81 mg	sulfur	56.7 mg

40 POINTS - THE BENEFITS OF WHEATGRASS JUICE

Note: All the following are cited from works of other authors and researchers listed under medical references.

1. Wheatgrass juice is one of the best sources of living chlorophyll available.

2. Chlorophyll is the first product of light and, therefore, contains more of the potential energy contained in light than any other molecule.

3. Wheatgrass juice is a crude chlorophyll and can be taken orally and as a colon implant without toxic side effects. To get the full benefit of chlorophyll it must be from a living plant and ingested within 6 minutes after juicing. [18]

4. Chlorophyll is the basis of all plant life.

5. Wheatgrass is high in oxygen like all green plants that contain chlorophyll. The brain and all body tissues function at an optimal level in a highly-oxygenated environment.

6. Chlorophyll is anti-bacterial and can be used inside and outside the body as a healer. [15, 16, 18, 19, 20, 21, 22, 24, 25, 36, 37, 40]

7. Dr. Bernard Jensen says that it only takes minutes to digest wheatgrass juice and uses up very little body energy.

8. Science has proven that chlorophyll arrests growth and development of unfriendly bacteria. [41]

9. Chlorophyll (wheatgrass) rebuilds the bloodstream. Studies of various animals have shown chlorophyll to be free of any toxic reaction. The red cell count was returned to normal within four to five days after the administration of chlorophyll, even in those animals

which were known to be extremely anemic or low in red cell count. [2, 23]

10. Farmers in the midwest who have sterile cows and bulls put them on wheatgrass to restore fertility. (The high magnesium content in chlorophyll builds enzymes that restore the sex hormones.) [11, 13]

11. Chlorophyll can be extracted from many plants, but wheatgrass is superior because it has been found to have over 100 elements needed by man. If grown in organic soil, it absorbs 92 of the known 102 minerals from the soil.

12. Wheatgrass has what is called the grass-juice factor, which has been shown to keep herbivorous animals alive indefinitely. [4, 8, 10]

13. Dr. Ann Wigmore has been helping people get well from chronic disorders for thirty years using wheatgrass.

14. Liquid chlorophyll gets into the tissues, vitalizes and refines them.

15. Wheatgrass juice is a superior detoxification agent compared to carrot juice and other fruits and vegetables. Dr. Earp-Thomas, associate of Ann Wigmore, says that 15 pounds of wheatgrass is the equivalent of 350 pounds of carrot, lettuce, celery, and so forth.

16. Liquid chlorophyll washes drug deposits from the body.

17. Chlorophyll neutralizes toxins in the body.

18. Chlorophyll helps purify the liver. [5, 27]

19. Chlorophyll improves blood sugar problems.

20. In the American Journal of Surgery (1940), Benjamin Gruskin, M.D. recommends chlorophyll for its antiseptic benefits. The article suggests the following clinical uses for chlorophyll: to clear up foul smelling odors, neutralize strep infections, heal wounds, hasten skin grafting, cure chronic sinusitis, overcome chronic inner-ear inflammation and infection, reduce varicose veins and heal leg ulcers, eliminate impetigo and other scabby eruptions, heal rectal sores, successfully treat inflammation of the uterine cervix, get rid of parasitic vaginal infections, reduce typhoid fever, and cure advanced pyorrhea in many cases.

21. Wheatgrass juice cures acne and even removes scars after it has been ingested for seven to eight months. The diet must be improved at the same time. [37]

22. Wheatgrass juice acts as a detergent in the body and is used as a body deodorant.

23. A small amount of wheatgrass juice in the human diet prevents tooth decay.

24. Wheatgrass juice held in the mouth for five to fiteen minutes will eliminate toothaches. It pulls poisons from the gums. [32,33]

25. Gargle wheatgrass juice for a sore throat.

26. Drink wheatgrass juice for skin problems such as eczema or psoriasis.

27. wheatgrass juice keeps the hair from graying.

28. To cure pyorrhea of the mouth lay pulp of wheatgrass soaked in juice on diseased area in mouth or chew wheatgrass, spitting out the pulp. [32, 33]

29. By taking wheatgrass juice, one may feel a difference in strength, endurance, health, and spirituality, and experience a sense of well being.

30. Wheatgrass juice improves the digestion.

31. Wheatgrass juice is high in enzymes.

32. Wheatgrass juice is an excellent skin cleanser and can be absorbed through the skin for nutrition. Pour green juice over your body in a tub of warm water and soak for fifteen to twenty minutes. Rinse off with cold water.

33. Wheatgrass implants (enemas) are great for healing and detoxifying the colon walls. The implants also heal and cleanse the internal organs. After an enema, wait twenty minutes, then implant 4 ounces of wheatgrass juice. Retain for twenty minutes. [18]

34. Wheatgrass juice is great for constipation and keeping the bowels open. It is high in magnesium. [18]

35. Dr. Birscher, a research scientist, called chlorophyll "concentrated sun power." He said, "chlorophyll increases the function of the heart, affects the vascular system, the intestines, the uterus, and the lungs."

36. According to Dr. Birscher, nature uses chlorophyll (wheatgrass) as a body cleanser, rebuilder, and neutralizer of toxins.

37. Wheatgrass juice can dissolve the scars that are formed in the lungs from breathing acid gasses. The effect of carbon monoxide is minimized since chlorophyll increases hemoglobin production. [1]

38. Wheatgrass Juice reduces high blood pressure and enhances the capillaries.

39. Wheatgrass Juice can remove heavy metals from the body.

40. Wheatgrass juice is great for blood disorders of all kinds.

MEDICAL REFERENCES - CHLOROPHYLL, CEREAL GRASSES

1. Hughes and Letner. "Chlorophyll and Hemoglobin Regeneration," American Journal of Medical Science. 188, 206 (1936)

2. Patek. "Chlorophyll and Regeneration of Blood." Archives of Internal Medicine. 57, 76 (1936)

3. Kohler, Elvahjem and Hart. "Growth Stimulating Properties of Grass Juice." Science. 83, 445 (1936)

4. Kohler, Elvahjem and Hart. "The Relation of the Grass Juice Factor to Guinea Pig Nutrition." Journal of Nutrition. 15, 445 (1938)

5. Rhoads. "The Relation of Vitamin K to the Hemorrhagic Tendency in Obstructive Jaundice (Dehydrated Cereal Grass as the Source of Vitamin K)." Journal of Medicine. 112, 2259, (1939)

6. Waddall. "Effect of Vitamin K on the Clotting Time of the Prothrombin and the Blood (Dehydrated Cereal Grass as the Source of Vitamin K)." Journal of Medicine. 112, 2259 (1939)

7. Illingworth. "Hemorrhage in Jaundice (Use of Dehydrated Cereal Grass)." Lancet. 236, 1031 (1939)

8. Kohler, Randle and Wagner. "The Grass Juice Factor." Journal of Biological Chemistry. 128, 1w (1939)

9. Friedman and Friedman. "Gonadotropic Extracts from Green Leaves." American Journal of Physiology. 125, 486, (1939)

10. Randle, Sober and Kohler. "The Distribution of the Grass Juice Factor in Plant and Animal Materials." The Journal of Nutrition. 20, 459 (1940)

11. Gomez, Hartman and Dryden. "Influence of Oat Juice Extract Upon the Age of Sexual Maturity in Rats." The Journal of Dairy Science. 24, 507 (1941)

12. Miller. "Chlorophyll for Healing." Science News Letter. March 15, 171 (1941)

13. Gomez. "Further Evidence of the Existence and Specificity of an Orally Active Sex Maturity Factor(s) in Plant Juice Preparations." The Journal of Dairy Science. 25, 705 (1942)

14. Kohler. "The Effect of Stage of Growth on the Chemistry of the Grasses." The Journal of Biological Chemistry. 215-23 (1944)

15. Boehme. "The Treatment of Chronic Leg Ulcers with Special Reference to Ointment Containing Water Soluble Chlorophyll." Cahey Clinical Bulletin. 4, 242 (1946)

16. Bowers. "Chlorophyll in Wound Healing and Suppurative Disease." The American Journal of Surgery. 71, 37 (1947)

17. Colio and Babb. "Study of a New Stimulatory Growth Factor," Journal of Biological Chemistry. 174, 405 (1948)

18. Juul-Moller and Middelsen. "Treatment of Intestinal Disease with Solutions of Water Soluble Chlorophyll." The Review of Gastroenterology. 15, 549 (1948)

19. Carpenter. "Clinical Experiences with Chlorophyll Preparations with Particular Reference to Chronic Osteomyelitis and Chronic Ulcer." American Journal of Surgery. 77, 267 (1949)

20. Offenkrantz. "Water-Soluble Chlorophyll in Ulcers of Long Duration." Review of Gastroenterology. 17, 359-67 (1950)

21. Anselmi. "Clinical Use of Chlorophyll and Derivatives." Minerva Medica. 2, 1313-14 (1950)

22. Lam and Brush. "Chlorophyll and Wound Healing: Experimental and Clinical Sudy." American Journal of Surgery. 80, 204-20 (1950)

23. Granick. "Structural and Functional Relationships between Heme and Chlorophyll." The Harvey Lectures. (1943-l949)

24. Cheney. "Antipeptic Ulcer Dietary Factor." The Journal of the American Dietetic Association. 26, 668 (1950)

25. Cheney. "The Nature of the Antipeptic Ulcer Factor." Stanford Medical Bulletin. 8, 144 (1950)

26. Sonsky. "Vitamin K Influence of Preventative Prenatal Administration." Ceskolovenska Gyneakologia. 29, 197 (1950)

27. Mossberg. "Vitamin K Treatment of Acute Hepatitus." British Medical Journal. 1, 1382-84 (1961)

28. Reid. "Treatment of Hypoprothrombinemia with Orally Administered Vitamin K." Quarterly Bulletin: Northwestern University Medical School. 25, 292-95 (1951)

29. Dohan, Richardson, Stribley and Gyorgy. "The Estrogenic Effects of Extracts of Spring Rye Grass." Journal of the American Veterinary Medicine Association. 118, 323 (1951)

30. Kohler and Graham. "A Chick Growth Factor Found in Leafy Green Vegetation," Poultry Science. 30, 484 (1951)

31. Paloscia and Pallotta. "Chlorophyll in Therapy." Lotta Controlla Tubercolosi. 22, 738-40 (1952)

32. Shattan and Kutcher. "Effect of Chlorophyll on Postextraction Healing." Journal of Oral Surgery. 46, 324 (1952)

33. Kutcher and Chilton. "Clinical Use of Chlorophyll Dentifrice." Journal of the American Dental Association. 46, 420-22 (1953)

34. Kohler. "The Unidentified Vitamins of Grass and Alfalfa." Feedstuffs Magazine. August 8 (1953).

35. Dunham. "Differential Inhibition of Virus Hemagglutination by Clorophyllin." Proceedings of the Society for Experimental Biology and Medicine. 87, 431-33 (1954)

36. Gandolfi. "Repitelizing Potency Exerted on Cornea by Chlorophyll." Annali de Ottalmologiale Clinica Oculistica. 80, 131-42 (1954)

37. Borelli. "Chlorophyll (for Acne Therapy)." Der Hautarzt. 6, 120-24 (1955)

38. Gandolfo. "Antismotic Activity of Chlorophyllin." Rendiconti Instituto Superiore de Sanita. 18, 641-48 (1955)

39. Offenkrantz. "Complete Healing (Peptic Ulcer) with Water-Soluble Chlorophyll." American Journal of Gastroenterology. 24, 182-85 (1955)

40. Wennig. "Modification and Inhibition of Resorption of Urinary Substances with Chlorophyllin." Wiener Medizinishe Wochenschrift. 105, 885-87 (1955)

41. Ammon and Wolfe. "Does Chloro;hyll have Bactericidal and Bacteriostatic Activity?" Arzneimettel-Forschung. 5, 312-14 (1955)

42. Bertram and Weinstock. "A Clinical Evaluation of Chlorophyll, Benzocain and Urea Ointment in Treatment of Minor Infections of the Foot." Journal of the American Podiatry Association. 19, 366 (1959)

THE MIRACLE OF GERMINATION

During germination, seeds become alive and undergo vast internal changes. And the great miracle of this amazing process is a huge increase in a host of nutrients which are miraculously created inside the sprouting embryo.

Water absorption swells the sprouting seed from six to ten times its normal size, creating tremendous dynamic pressures per square inch. Enzymes immediately become active and create a host of nutritional changes. Chlorophyll and carotene content increase dramatically when they are exposed to sunlight.

Wheat sprouts for example, contain four times more folic acid and six times more vitamin C than unsprouted wheat. In studies at the University of Pennsylvania, vitamin C content in some seeds was found to increase up to 700 percent in just the first seventy two hours of sprouting! For this reason, some fresh sprouts contain more vitamin C than citrus juices. This also applies to vitamins A, E, the B complex and others, depending on the variety of seed sprouted. A Yale University study of grains, seeds, and beans showed that sprouting substantially increases all B-vitamins from 20 percent to 600 percent. Vitamin E content increases 300 percent in sprouted wheat after four days of sprouting.

Sprouts are complete foods. Their proteins are called "complete proteins" because in correct combinations they contain all the essential amino acids. They are also called "complete foods" because they contain all other essential dietary nutrients, along with enzymes to help assimilate them. Simple plant sugars such as maltose are easily digested and enter the bloodstream quickly. For this reason, sprouts are also classed as "quick-energy" foods. Sprouts are live foods because they are living plants. This means that sprouts have living protein versus the dead protein found in animal foods. Let's take a closer look at several of the most delicious and nutritious sprouts.

Sprouted wheat that grows into wheatgrass about 8 inches long is a potent source of concentrated nutrition. As it grows, wheatgrass concentrates chlorophyll and other nutrients in preparation for becoming a big, fruitful plant. Wheatgrass itself is not digestible in our stomachs because it is too full of cellulose and other indigestible fibers. But when juiced and strained, all the nutrients are freed and are readily assimilable by the body.

Wheatgrass juice is a very powerful body detoxifier. Its high chlorophyll content cleanses the liver, tissues and cells and purifies the blood. Placed in the nose, a few drops can reduce inflamed nasal passages and sinuses, relieving congestion without chemicals. Gargling will help relieve a sore throat. Wheatgrass juice is an excellent natural mouthwash and breath deodorizer. It will leave the breath smelling naturally fresh while nutrifying the gums and delicate tissues of the mouth. Some have used it on the skin to relieve pain and skin problems.

GROWING WHEATGRASS OR BARLEY GRASS

This method is used for growing wheatgrass, barley grass, or other similar grasses for juicing. It requires a few special materials. You will need to begin with:

- 2 cups (1 lb) of hard red winter or spring wheat or unhulled barley seeds
- 1 gallon jar or large bowl for soaking seeds
- Tray, roughly 10" x 21" x 2"
- Soil to cover seedling tray 1-inch deep. Use sifted forest mulch from a nursery—organic is the safest and best
- It is best to use a seedling tray with holes as grass grows better with good drainage

- Soil amendment such as Azomite™ to dust planting surface
- Watering can equipped with sprinkler head
- 4 to 5 layers of paper towels or empty tray to cover growing tray
- Spray bottle
- Serrated knife
- Wheatgrass juicer

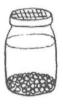

Step One: Simply soak the seeds or grain overnight for six to eight hours. Be sure seeds are fully immersed, with an extra couple of inches of water over the top. After soaking about six hours, pour off water, rinse, leave in container and let sprout for another six to ten hours.

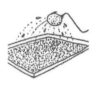

Step Two: Spread soil mixture evenly on seedling tray about 1-inch deep and pack lightly. Sprinkle a light dusting of Azomite™ over the prepared soil bed. Lightly moisten the soil with the gentle, even spray of the sprinkler watering can. Don't overdo it—make no puddles. Spread the soaked seeds evenly over the surface of the soil only one layer thick.

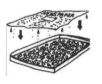

Step Three: Cover the seeds with four to five layers of paper towels and wet them, or invert an empty tray over the growing tray. If you use the inverted tray, be sure the soil has been moistened, but not over watered. Set tray in a cool (but not cold), dark place away from temperature extremes or drafts.

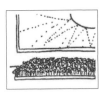

Step Four: Water the paper towels to make sure the paper is not drying out. If dry, use a spray bottle mister to lightly redampen it. If you see evidence of mold, wipe it off and find a cooler spot (mold indicates too much heat and moisture). You can lightly spray the mold with a solution of 1 tablespoon Real Salt in ½ gallon of water. Use your spray bottle.

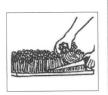

Step Five: When grass blades are about 1-inch high (in about three days), remove the paper towels gently and expose the grass to light. From now on, water once per day until water drips from bottom of tray.

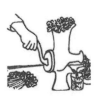

Step Six: When 3 to 4 inches tall, continue to expose to indirect sunlight each day. A cool breeze is helpful during sunning to keep the grass from overheating, or use a fan near the tray on low speed. During inclement weather, use a plant growing light or LED light for three to four hours each day instead.

Step Seven: Harvest with a serrated knife or scissors when 6 to 8 inches tall. Grasp a bunch and cut about ½-inch above the soil. Sunflower, buckwheat and fenugreek can be used directly in salads or juiced. Wheatgrass, because of its high cellulose content, will have to be juiced. If the grass has mold, power rinse!

Step Eight: Grind the cut grass in a juicer and strain. The best juicers turn at a slow speed (around 80 rpm), are made of stainless steel or a very heavy food grade plastic (avoid aluminum) and are built to last. Blenders spin too fast and can oxidize enzymes.

Wheatgrass juice is best taken right after juicing for highest nutritional content. You can refrigerate for a day or two if you use an airtight jar, and some promote storing the juice before using because over a period of six to eight hours, the abscissic acid content of the juice will increase significantly. It will keep for a longer period if frozen quickly right after juicing. Wheatgrass juice can be a real tonic for the body because it is high in all the antioxidants, enzymes, and simple sugars for quick energy. Ann Wigmore recommended drinking the juice within six minutes after juicing for best results. If you have never drunk wheatgrass juice, begin with only 1 ounce per day. Gradually build to 2 ounces per day.

A normal juicing would yield 2 ounces of juice, which should be taken within six minutes of juicing. Some people juice twice per day. Each 10" x 21" tray generally yields about 12 to 14 ounces of juice, so you can figure that you will use one tray per week per person.

COCOTEK® GROWING INSTRUCTIONS:
FOR WHEATGRASS, BARLEY GRASS, BUCKWHEAT GREENS, AND SUNFLOWER GREENS.

1. Place the CocoTek mat into the black tray with no holes. Cover with salt water (2 tablespoons salt). Soak 2 hours. Rinse the mat well. (Later the tray with no holes can be used under the tray with holes to protect your furniture.)

2. Put the CocoTek mat into a black tray with holes. Sprinkle one handful of Azomite™ over the mat, evenly. Azomite™ is a trace mineral that ensures the highest nutritional value of your sprouted grass.

3. Rinse one package of seed two or three times before you soak. Place one package of pre-measured (2 cups) wheatgrass or barley grass seed into a jar and fill the jar with water so that water completely immerses the seed. Soak the seed overnight (eight to twelve hours in the winter and six to eight hours in the summer. Soak in refrigerator during hot part of summer).

4. Drain off the water, and rinse the seed well. Plant the seed anytime during the day, spreading them evenly over the coco mat in a thick layer to ensure abundant juice.

5. Cover the seed with about four layers of dry paper towels. Spray water directly over the paper towels until the towels and the seed and mat beneath are soaked thoroughly, and the water drips from the bottom of the tray.

6. For the next three days, keep newspaper or paper towel wet! Important! If newspaper dries out, the root hairs on the sprouts will dry out and the grass will not come up well. A piece of plastic can be laid over

the newspaper to keep it from drying out too quickly. On the second or third day take the newspaper off and water the grass and then place the newspaper back on for one more day. (In 1936 the United States Government mandated that all newsprint ink be made with vegetable oil. It is completely non toxic.) If you have a compost pile, it is good to add this newspaper to the pile. It adds carbon and sweetens your compost.

7. When the grass is 1 to 2 inches tall, remove the paper and expose to indirect light. If it is extremely hot outside, put the tray in the shade. If you grow it inside the house, drain over your sink when you water, and then place the grass near a window. A cool but sunny place is ideal.

8. Water your wheat or barley grass two or three times per day until it drips from the bottom. (If you live in an extremely dry climate, it would be a good idea to water once per day even while the seed is under the paper.)

9. Keep your wheat in a cool place with moving air if possible. Sometimes in hotter climates wheatgrass and barley grass will show signs of mold near the roots. If you have problems with mold, cut what you are going to juice, put it in a big strainer or colander and power rinse the grass very well before you juice. Sometimes this will help eliminate the mold: Get some Real Salt from your health food store. Use 1 tablespoon per ½ gallon water. Wash with this solution once after removing the paper. If all else fails, we have a product called Mold Control on our website.

10. Harvest the grass when it is six to seven inches tall. You can harvest only what you are going to juice at

that time or you can harvest the whole tray. If you harvest the whole tray, put it in a plastic bag and store in your refrigerator. The grass will stay fresh in the refrigerator. When the weather is cooler, it is better to harvest as you juice. (If you have room, the whole tray can be put in the refrigerator.)

11. It takes very little wheatgrass per day to satisfy the nutritional needs of a normal person. One ounce is a good start if you have never had wheatgrass juice before. Gradually increase you daily intake until you find the amount with which you are comfortable. A typical person should increase the amount of grass juice they take by one ounce every two or three weeks up to a total of 4 ounces. Some people choose to remain at 2 ounces.

Each tray of 6 to 7-inch-tall grass will yield approximately 12 ounces of juice. Depending upon the amount you use, you will probably need to space your planting every five to six days and as you gradually use more, plant every three to four days.

Also we do not recommend re-using the mats for a second crop.

MOLD

Wheatgrass is sometimes susceptible to mold. To control the mold here are a few steps you can take:

1. Soak your seed from six to eight hours. In the summer, only soak six hours. Rinse the seed extremely well before and after soaking.

2. Water once with Real (Mineral) Salt, or Azomite™ when the wheatgrass is very young (right after uncovering). Use 1 tablespoon per ½ gallon. The silicates in the Azomite™ and in the mineral salt will cut right through the mold.

3. Keep the growing temperature somewhat cool (70 degrees) and also dry.

4. If you still have problems with mold simply put the grass into a big strainer or colander and power rinse the grass very well before you juice it.

5. Ventilation is important. Direct a slow fan towards your grass after you uncover.

6. Using the LED light solves mold problems also in that the ultra-violet light from the LED light eradicates most mold. In addition to solving your mold problems, the LED light will turn your grass a deep, dark green and it will stay green longer.

7. You can add a capful of hydrogen peroxide to the soaking water to help control for mold.

8. Be sure to remove any "floaters", seeds which are broken or are still floating twenty minutes after you have started the soaking process.

9. You can use a few drops of grapefruit seed extract (in glycerin) in the soaking water.

10. You can spray the wheatgrass with a mild hydrogen peroxide solution (one small capful in a spray bottle filled with water).

11. You can place the moldy tray in direct sunlight for a short period of time after spraying with a salt or peroxide solution.

Mold can be a real problem in warmer weather, or when you grow inside your home in the winter and it is warm and humid. Be scrupulously clean, and be sure to clean trays very well between plantings. You may use the grass when there is evidence of mold, but you should be sure to rinse it very well, and inspect it closely before juicing.

IDEAL WEATHER

If it is too cold outside (50 degrees and below) where you are growing your grass, the wheatgrass will grow very slowly. If you let it get below 32 degrees, it will freeze. Anything above about 75 to 80 degrees and your wheatgrass will not thrive. Under the hot conditions you will experience more mold, and the roots will go sour and sometimes cause the grass to wilt. The ideal conditions for wheatgrass and barley grass are 1) indirect sunlight, and 2) moderate weather (70 degrees).

GROWING SPACE

Space often can become a problem once you start growing lots of wheatgrass and sprouts. Very inexpensive racks can be purchased from a local hardware store, or you can make a rack with PVC pipes. This seems to be a better solution for those who have their wheatgrass scattered all over their kitchen. Growing racks with and without full spectrum lights can be found at www.wheatgrasskits.com.

OLD GRASS

If you don't use the grass fast enough, your wheatgrass will get old, so here is a good solution. Whether you buy or grow your own flat of wheatgrass, if you don't use the grass fast enough it begins to turn yellow and wilt (because it has used all the minerals from the soil). Right as it begins to tinge yellow, cut all the rest of the grass off of the flat and put it in a plastic bag in your refrigerator. The grass will last for about one week after it is cut. Using an inexpensive LED light will keep your grass from turning yellow so fast.

MICROGREENS

Microgreens are an entirely individual crop of their own. They are tiny, thin immature plants and are grown to be small—in fact the smallest sprinkling of herbs, edible flowers salad greens, and leafy vegetables. One can grow almost any seed and call it a microgreen, however there are some varieties that have been proven to be superior because of their unique shape, flavor and color and micro size.

They are grown in different kinds of mediums, from what is called a baby bud blanket, to peat moss, to a coco fibre mat. Microgreens make a one-time harvest and are clipped one time at the surface of the soil or growing medium as soon as their true leaves appear. The difference between sprouts and microgreens is that sprouts are not grown in a medium and their roots are eaten along with the sprout, whereas microgreens are clipped right above the root. Shoots, such as sunflower greens, peas, and buckwheat greens are also clipped at the bottom of the stem, however they are a little larger than the micro-greens. organicmicro-greens.com has developed a starter kit to help you begin to grow and utilize these greens and to simplify your growing experience. Superior micro-green seed combinations are available to make it easy and delicious to get started.

Instructions: Soak your seed mixture for seven to nine hours. Get a 10 by 20 inch seedling flat with holes. Put into the bottom of the tray about an inch of the growing medium (organic potting mixture, bud blanket, or peat moss). Sprinkle the seeds evenly over the surface of the soil and gently press the seeds into the soil. Cover the seeds with three to four layers of paper towels and water the paper towels until the water drips from the bottom of the tray. (Important! Keep the paper towels wet until the micro-greens are at least one inch tall.) Another option: put a clear plastic dome over the seeds after planting.

When the plants are about one inch tall, remove the paper towels (you can leave the plastic dome on if used) and expose to light. You can place the tray under a grow light, outdoors in the shade or by a warm (not hot) window. When the first true leaves appear, they are ready to harvest (this is usually about ten days after planting). Clip the stems right above the growing medium. Put greens in a large colander, gently rinse. You can then either put into a salad spinner if you have one, or you can lay out to dry on a regular towel. Store either in a mason jar or in plastic bags in your fridge. If you have grown them on soil, you can just leave them growing and clip them as you need them.

These tiny gourmet nutritious vegetables are served in trendy restaurants around the world. They provide a colorful and healthy addition to any dish.

WHAT VARIETIES OF VEGETABLES SHOULD YOU USE?

Many different types are grown in this way such as arugula, a mildly spicy member of the brassica family. Broccoli is good as it is known for its anti-oxidant properties. Other options are green and red cabbage varieties, oriental cabbages, kohlrabi, swiss chard, radish, beetroot, and red kale, edamame, petite fava, cucumber, horseradish, micro-mint, lavender, herb mixes, amaranth, pepper grass, giant red mustard, red radish, and wrinkled cress. These are just a few of the micro-greens that can be grown and eaten right in your own kitchen.

Microgreens can be grown any time of the year—even inside during winter. For use in the house you can buy special felt pads on which you grow the seeds instead of soil. Each crop takes between two to three weeks from sowing the seeds until they are ready for harvesting.

For unusual salads and to add to cooking, mirco-greens can spice up your cuisine. Microgreens with a strong pungent taste can be added to salads to give it more taste. Some have unusual flavours which add much interest to your soups, salads, and cooking. Hopefully this brief introduction to microgreens has given you some ideas, and perhaps will encourage you to try growing a crop yourself.

GROWING SUNFLOWER AND BUCKWHEAT GREENS

Along with wheatgrass juice and sprouts, freshly harvested greens are an excellent addition to the diet. The two most nutritious and easily grown greens are sunflower and buckwheat.

When growing these types of greens you should use soil, and in both cases, unhulled seed. Greens, in conjunction with sprouts and wheatgrass juice, represent the most complete source of chlorophyll-rich food to go along with fermented foods in the Wigmore diet.

This method is used for sprouting sunflower and buckwheat, and requires a few special materials. It is almost identical to growing wheatgrass.

Often, you will split a single 10" x 21" tray between the two types of seeds. You can use the same growing materials as you would with wheatgrass, and generally the same growing conditions and time frames.

You will need to begin with:

- 1 cup each of sunflower and buckwheat seeds
- 1 gallon jar or large bowl for soaking seeds separately
- Tray, roughly 10" x 21"
- Soil to cover seedling tray 1 inch deep. Use sifted forest mulch from a nursery—organic if they have it
- Watering can equipped with sprinkler head
- Four to five layers of paper towel or empty tray to cover growing tray
- Spray bottle
- Serrated knife or scissors

Step One: Simply soak the seeds overnight for six to eight hours. Be sure seeds are fully immersed, with an extra couple of inches of water over the top. After soaking six hours, pour off water, rinse, leave in soaking container and let sprout for another six to ten hours.

Step Two: Spread soil mixture evenly on seedling tray about 1-inch deep and pack lightly. Sprinkle a light dusting of Azomite™ over the prepared soil bed. Lightly moisten the soil with the gentle, even spray of the sprinkler watering can. Don't overdo it—make no puddles. Spread the soaked seeds evenly over the surface of the soil only one layer thick.

Step Three: Cover the seeds with four to five layers of paper towel cut to the size of the tray, or invert an empty tray over the growing tray. Set tray in a cool (but not cold), dark place away from temperature extremes or drafts. Wet the paper towels.

Step Four: Raise the tray or paper towels once a day to give them fresh air and to make sure the paper is not drying out. If dry, use the mister to lightly redampen it. If you see evidence of mold, wipe it off and find a cooler spot (mold indicates too much heat and moisture). You can lightly spray the mold with a solution of 1 teaspoon sea (or real) salt in ½ gallon of water. Use your spray bottle.

Step Five: When greens are about 1-inch high (in about three days), remove the paper towels gently and expose them to indirect light. From this point on, water once per day until water drips from bottom.

Step Six: Continue to expose to indirect sunlight each day, A cool breeze is helpful during sunning to keep the greens from overheating, or use a fan near the tray on low speed. During inclement weather, use a plant growing light or LED lights for three to four hours each day instead.

Step Seven: Harvest with a serrated knife or scissors when 4 to 6 inches tall. Grasp a bunch and cut about ½ to 1 inch above the soil. Sunflower, buckwheat and fenugreek can be used directly in salads or juiced. You can refrigerate several days in a plastic bag.

HULL REMOVAL

One of the chores associated with growing seeds that have hulls is removing those that do not fall off of their own accord. As the tray matures, you can pluck off hulls ready to drop to reduce the amount of handling when you harvest. It is also useful to have a mat or something on the floor below the greens tray to catch the hulls as they drop off over the growing period.

Some folks have used a small hand held mini-vacuum to gently vacuum off the hulls, but this is a bit tricky until you get the hang of it.

MOLD

Review the section on wheatgrass and mold to learn about techniques to control for this.

RESULTS

Dr. Wigmore claimed that you could easily feed a family of four from your indoor garden using organic seed grown or sprouted under your own close supervision. In this way you not only save money, but you insure your family that their food was of the highest quality, freshness, and nutritional value. The fact that you know it is free of chemicals and pathogens, and that this diet is the most environmentally sensitive, makes it an all around winner.

Dr. Wigmore claimed that sunflower greens were a great protein addition to the diet, and that buckwheat greens very specifically helped the circulatory system due to their high rutin and lecithin content. She recommended using the cut greens in salads, raw soups, and on their own.

SPROUTS AND GOOD HEALTH

Alfalfa Sprouts - One of the most popular, nutritious and delicious of all sprouting seeds. High in protein, essential amino acids, and eight digestive enzymes; vitamins A, C, B complex (including B-12), D, E, and 4 minerals; iron, phosphorous, calcium, magnesium, and potassium, and, when exposed to light, high in chlorophyll. Alfalfa sprouts are very tasty, with a sweet, nut-like flavor. They are a lot safer, less expensive, and more fun to eat than factory-field, chemicalized lettuce. Alfalfa seeds sprout easily in combination with other seeds. They make a lively addition to the diet in salads, sandwiches, soups etc.

Barley *(unhulled organic)* - Barley grass, much like wheatgrass, is rich in B vitamins particularly thiamine, riboflavin, protein and many minerals. Barley has an extremely high content of organic sodium. People who tend to be arthritic need organic sodium and do much better with barley rather than wheatgrass. Soak the unhulled grain overnight and place close together in a tray of sifted organic forest mulch (from any nursery). Cover with wet paper after watering the entire tray and block light for three to four days with black plastic. Expose to light for additional three to four days and continue to water as needed. Cut 1 inch from base to harvest and juice in a slow revolution juicer. Delicious and nutritious!

Broccoli Sprouts *(raw)* - Provide vitamins A, B, C; potassium and the phytochemicals sulforaphane; indole and isothiocyanate. Research suggests these phytochemicals may reduce the risk of breast, stomach, and lung cancers.

Buckwheat Sprouts - Rich in protein, iron, calcium, phosphorous, vitamin B complex, vitamin E and large amounts of rutin and bioflavonoids. Rutic acid has a powerful beneficial effect on the arteries and circulatory system. Bioflavonoids work with vitamin C to help detox the body and build the immune system. Buckwheat lettuce makes a tasty addition to any salad.

Chinese Cabbage Sprouts - Provide lots of vitamin A and C, minerals, and when exposed to light are high in chlorophyll as well. They even taste like cabbage and are excellent when chopped up in cole slaw. Do not sprout for too long (see sprouting chart on page 46) or they will taste bitter.

Fenugreek Sprouts - Contain choline (a fat controller) and are rich in protein, iron, and vitamins A, D and G. Fenugreek is a strongly scented herb of the pea family. It is reported to be helpful for digestive problems including ulcers. It is spicy and a major component in curry powder. These sprouts are best used sparingly in salads, soups, sandwiches, curries and rice dishes. Also acts as an herb for dissolving mucus in the body when taken as a tea. These sprouts are said to be good for breastfeeding moms because they help with milk production.

Garbanzo - Rich in carbohydrates, fiber, calcium and protein as well as magnesium, potassium and vitamins A and C. Soak eight hours, rinse and drain. Spread evenly in sprouter. Rinse two to three times per day for three to four days. Do not expose to sunlight. Garbanzo makes an enzyme rich hummus when sprouted one to two days and mixed in a blender.

Soybean - A very versatile bean that can lower cholesterol and protect against cancer through its healthy protease inhibitors. Good for keeping blood sugar under control. Great in salads, stir frys, soups and breads. Use the same methods to sprout as green pea and garbanzo.

Sunflower Sprouts - High in fiber, protein, essential fatty acids, vitamins A, B complex, C, D, and E. They also contain calcium, phosphorous, iron, iodine, potassium, magnesium and the trace elements zinc, manganese, copper and chromium. Sunflower sprouts taste like nothing else you have ever tasted, with a flavor all their own.

Green Pea - Rich in chlorophyll, protein, enzymes and minerals. Whole peas would be sprouted using the above method for two to three days. Do not expose to light.

Lentil Sprouts - High in fiber, protein and amino acids, vitamins A, C, B complex and E, iron, calcium and phosphorus. Raw lentil sprouts can be a bit peppery to the taste. Their flavor is more sweet and nut-like when cooked. Lentils sprout well with other seeds. They make a good substitute for celery or green pepper in salads, soups and vegetable combinations. Sprouted lentil soup is hearty and nutritious and was a staple food of the middle east in biblical times.

Mung Bean Sprouts - Another nutritional powerhouse. High in choline protein and the amino acid methionine vitamins A, B complex C and E; minerals calcium, magnesium, potassium, and phosphorous; trace elements zinc, chromium, iron. Mung bean sprouts have a crisp, crunchy texture and a flavor similar to fresh-picked garden peas. They are a tasty addition to salads, vegetable dishes and oriental main dishes.

Radish Sprouts - High in vitamins, A, B-1, B-6, and C, folic and pantothenic acids, niacin, potassium, iron and phosphorous. When exposed to light, they turn light green with chlorophyll. Radish sprouts are crisp, slightly hot and tangy, like tiny radishes. They sprout well with other seeds and make a spicy addition to any vegetable dish.

Red Clover Sprouts - Resemble alfalfa sprouts and contain many of the same vitamins, minerals and amino acids. They also turn green with chlorophyll when exposed to light. They add a zestful taste to salads and other dishes and sprout well with other seeds.

Red Winter Wheat Sprouts - Probably the most nutritious, delicious and versatile of all the sprouted grains. High in fiber, protein, amino acids, vitamins A, C, B complex and E, niacin and panthothenic acid. Sprouted wheat is full of the sugar maltose and has a sweet, nutty flavor. It can be used in a wide variety of ways, including sprouted wheat breads and for making wheatgrass juice.

THE LIVING FOOD DIET
AS TAUGHT BY ANN WIGMORE
by KK Fowlkes

Many people have asked: What specifically is the living food diet which was taught by Ann Wigmore? Briefly I will explain the diet without going into too much information about the Ann Wigmore Foundation which is now located in San Fidel, New Mexico.

Ann Wigmore, pioneer of the living food wheatgrass diet, wrote about 35 books during her lifetime in which one can find out more about her. Some titles I suggest are, *Why Suffer, Be Your Own Doctor, Hippocrates Diet and Health Program, The Wheatgrass Book, and The Sprouting Book.* The last book written before her death was A Scientific Appraisal of Dr. Ann Wigmore's Living Foods Lifestyle. A book that further explains why her diet works is Enzyme Nutrition by Edward Howell.

Basically, in simple terms, the diet (which includes wheatgrass juice) restores the body's vitality such as the body's ability to heal itself. Just as the body has the ability to heal a cut or a bruise, it should also have the ability to heal a cancer or an arthritic condition or any number of illnesses. Why has the body lost its vitality? Cooked food. Dead food. If food is eaten which has the life force intact (raw, sprouted) then the life force in the food transfers into the life force of the body.

The instruction at the institute covers these areas:

- Diet (living, raw)
- Wheatgrass juice
- Bowel rejuvenation
- Exercise

When I attended Ann Wigmore's Institute in Boston many years ago, I noticed that she kept the diet very simple. I feel that she did so, so as not to overwhelm people with an extensive array of foods and recipes which when they got home they thought they had to duplicate. Her different books cover a wider array of recipes if one is interested in more of a variety.

THE DIET

1. Fresh fruit or fresh pressed fruit juice for breakfast. Sometimes she would blend a mild sprout (hulled buckwheat) with fruit for a breakfast cereal. (Buckwheat sprouts are considered a fruit and have a high content of vitamin C.)

2. For lunch, a large sprouted salad consisting of buckwheat and sunflower greens, sprouted alfalfa and sprouted fenugreek with a dressing made from seed cheese and a bowl of energy soup.

3. Afternoon snack of fresh or dried fruit.

4. For dinner, another large salad containing sprouted sunflower, buckwheat, alfalfa, fenugreek with a seed cheese dressing with a bowl of energy soup. Sometimes include a sunflower seed cheese veggie loaf and veggie kraut.

5. Wheatgrass juice was always available as was a fermented wheat sprout drink called rejuvelac, which she recommended one drink instead of water. Rejuvelac adds enzymes to the diet as does the veggie kraut.

Condiments on the table included cayenne pepper, seed cheese salad dressing, and sometimes almond cream.

Her diet is revolutionary in that it is:

1. Incredibly inexpensive

2. A food

3. A medicine

4. A survival tool

In addition to strengthening the immune system to fight deadly microbes and curing major ailments, live chlorophyll cures radiation sickness. The manual wheatgrass juicer can be used to juice the grass in the field if no other food is available.

WHEATGRASS JUICE

Fresh pressed juice to be taken twice or three times per day on an empty stomach (one hour before a meal or two hours after). Amount should not exceed 1 ounce per day the first week or 2 ounces for extreme detoxifying properties. Gradually build up to 3 to 4 ounces. Sometime people who are extremely ill will build up to 4 ounces in the morning and 4 ounces at night.

BARLEY GRASS JUICE

Barley grass juice was not a part of Ann's diet. However some people use it instead of wheatgrass juice because it is high in organic sodium, is milder and can be used every day, month after month, without the body building up an aversion to it. Many people like to use it in the summer to replace sodium lost during heat.

BOWEL REJUVENATION

Bowel rejuvenation consists of water enemas and wheat-grass implants once or twice daily to assist the liver to detoxify. This is an area where you need to research how it is done, and exactly what techniques you need to master to accomplish cleansing safely.

EXERCISE

Exercise gently for the very ill. Ann Wigmore used mini trampolines. This exercise stimulates and increases circulation and helps the lymphatic system discharge toxins. Persons who are very ill should remain on the diet for at least eighteen months or longer.

WHY SPROUTING IS IDEAL

Besides their nutritional advantages, sprouted seeds, beans and grains have several other sterling attributes that make them an ideal addition to your regular diet and a prime food source in times of need. Sprouts are:

- Economical. One tablespoon of seeds, costing less than 50 cents, will fill a quart jar with several ounces of delicious, ready-to-eat sprouts. A 4-ounce package will yield several pounds. And this concentrated nutrition is alive. Something which can't be said for most nutritional supplements that cost much more.

- Ecological. Because they are such nutritional powerhouses, their food value is much higher than most other foods per unit of production cost. This conserves energy and saves processing, packaging and storage costs. And it avoids "denaturing" and toxic build-up in the food itself.

- Toxin-Free. Sprouts are as sweet and pure as nature intended food to be.

When completely natural and organic and sprouted with clean water, they can be free of toxic residues. Living Whole Foods distributors supply only natural, non-treated sprouting seeds with up to 99 percent rates of germination, grown especially for sprouting.

Caution: To prevent infestation and mold, seeds used for planting are treated with chemical pesticides, fungicides and mercury coatings that can be highly toxic. Imported seeds are required by law to be dyed for identification. Therefore, for your own protection, heed this warning:

CAUTIONARY

NEVER SPROUT SEEDS, BEANS, GRAINS ETC. THAT HAVE BEEN CHEMICALLY TREATED OR DYED. SPROUT ONLY THOSE SEEDS THAT HAVE BEEN EXPLICITLY CERTIFIED AS EDIBLE.

If you do get mold on your sprouting seed, it can be power rinsed, but inspect it closely to be sure all mold has been washed off. For this reason also, you should thoroughly clean all sprouting containers after each use, preferably in hot, soapy water with a scrub brush.

SPROUTING ADVANTAGES

Easy to Store - Seeds do not have to be frozen or pre-served to keep them from spoiling. All they require is a few glass jars with air-tight lids and a cool, dark storage area. They will store easily in very little space for a year or more. One small, lower shelf (heat rises, higher shelves are warmer) in a pantry will hold enough assorted seeds to feed an entire family for months. After sprouting, they can be placed in plastic bags in the refrigerator, again not requiring much space.

Low in Calories/Fat - Depending on protein content, one fully packed cup of sprouts contains only 16 to 70 calories. And these are simple sugars for quick energy. Sprouts contain no cholesterol and provide essential fatty acids. Several, such as alfalfa, are sweet and satisfying to the taste buds and the body. It is almost impossible to overeat raw live foods such as sprouts. They are the perfect weight-loss and body-purification food for the new millennium.

Tasty and Versatile - Bursting with flavor, you may be surprised how truly delectable they are. You can enjoy a wide variety of new taste sensations. Just add or substitute wherever you use vegetables. They take very little time to prepare when steamed, boiled, or stir-fried, cooked or even baked in wholesome, homemade breads. You will find several delicious, easy-to-prepare and satisfying recipe ideas at the end of this booklet.

Simple, Easy and Fast to Grow - This "garden in your hand" grows very fast in any weather with very little care. Most of them take less than a minute or two per day to grow. You can grow sprouts year round, nearly anywhere indoors in any season, without any weather worries. No digging, planting, weeding, pests or chemicals to worry about either, And no long wait, as in outdoor vegetable gardens. In just three to seven days, you will have a nutrition-packed, bountiful harvest. When stored in your refrigerator, they will stay fresh for days—even weeks if rinsed properly. Because they require very little space and travel well, sprouts are the ideal vegetables for campers, boaters and RV'ers. Complete, easy-to-follow instructions are given below and in the sprouting kits available from Living Whole Food distributors. Specific instructions for each variety of seeds or seed mix are provided on the back of every Living Whole Foods seed label.

HOW TO GROW SPROUTS

Good sprouting technique doesn't take a "green thumb," just paying attention to four factors: the right amount of moisture, the correct temperature, the free circulation of air, and minimal light. By rinsing them a couple of times daily, you keep them moist. You also wash away carbon dioxide and other metabolic wastes that could cause souring or spoiling. Using cool water when rinsing ventilates and cools the sprouts to prevent overheating. Proper draining prevents excessive moisture that can cause mold and rot. The ideal sprouting temperature depends on the seed, but generally lies between 70 degrees and 85 degrees fahrenheit (see sprouting chart on page 46). To protect the tiny growing things, keep sprouting containers away from cold drafts, direct heat, or any light. For free air circulation, at least one-third of the container must be empty. Sprouts expand 6 to 10 times over a few days, so give them plenty of room to grow. Sprouts are very light sensitive and need to be covered during the early stages of the growing cycle.

SIMPLE TECHNIQUES

- Rinse often.
- Keep them moist, not wet.
- Keep them at room temperature.
- Give them plenty of room to breathe.
- Don't put too many in any one container.
- Keep them covered—no light.
- Refrigerate after four days of sprouting on a counter top.

Sprouts will continue to grow slowly in the fridge, so rinse every two days after refrigerating.

Caution: Although bulk seeds, beans and grains may appear cheaper than Living Whole Food seeds, it may not be to your advantage to use them for sprouting. Unless they are packaged as high-germination sprouting seeds, only part of them may sprout. This means that some seeds may ferment and spoil the whole batch. You will have to pick out the unsprouted seeds one by one. Otherwise, any you leave in will add hard spots and a bitter taste to what should be a succulent mass of tender, tasty sprouts.

JAR METHOD

This is by far the oldest and most popular method as well as one of the easiest.

All you need is a standard wide mouth, threaded, quart, half-gallon or gallon glass jar. One technique is to cover the mouth of your sprouting jar with muslin, cheese cloth or nylon mesh screen. This will work, but the screen is subject to mold and mildew build-up and is not as easy as using special sprouting lids designed specifically for this purpose.

Living Whole Foods www.wheatgrasskits.com offers a number of jar sprouters in plastic and glass to choose from (seeds included), as well as the single polyethylene screen cap to add to your own wide mouth jar. Whatever the method or type used, the idea is to rinse away the unnecessary hulls for cleaner, fresher sprouts.

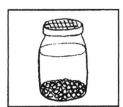

Step One: Soaking

For a quart-sized jar, start with 1 ½ tablespoons or more of seeds (see sprouting chart on page 46). Place the seeds you wish to sprout inside the jar, screw on the fine mesh lid and partially fill the jar with warm water, not hot. Swirl it around to clean the seeds, then pour it out. Now refill with warm water to cover the seeds about three times their depth and let the seeds soak three to four hours, or for the time indicated in the sprouting chart (page 46)during the day. To protect from light, keep jar covered or place in cabinet overnight.

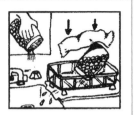

Step Two: Draining and Starting

Pour off the soak water. Find a location that is not exposed to direct sunlight. Place drained jar propped at an angle to allow any extra water to drain out. Turn the jar to spread out the seed. Cover the jar with a dish towel and leave for three to four hours.

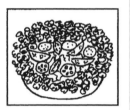

Step Three: Rinsing

Rinse the sprouts with cool, fresh water two or three times each day until they are ready to eat or refrigerate. When they begin to throw off the seed hulls, let the jar overflow with water and the hulls will float out the top through the screen. Turn the jar to spread out the seed each time you rinse.

Step Four: Harvesting

Pour the sprouts into a pan or sink of clean water. Skim off any remaining hulls that float to the surface. Other hulls will fall to the bottom of the container. A few stubborn hulls may have to be removed individually by hand. This does not apply to those, such as wheat berries, which have no hulls. Pull out the sprouts, gently shake off excess moisture and drain in a colander. When fully drained, either use them or place in a sealed, airtight container such as a reclosable plastic bag which leaves some room for air circulation.

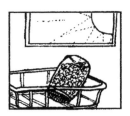

Step Five: Greening

Remove the sprouts and clean the jar and lid. Place sprouts for greening back into the jar. Place in indirect sunlight. Near a kitchen window is fine, After the sprouts have greened with chlorophyll and carotenes for a day or so, rinse, drain and eat or refrigerate.

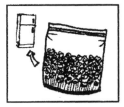

Step Six: Refrigerating

Refrigerate after 4 days!
For chlorophyll and carotene-developing sprouts, there is an added step, one day before the final harvest. Sprouts will stay fresh and hearty for a week or more when refrigerated, if you rinse them every day or two. You can even give the green sprouts an extra hour or two of sunlight after rinsing to keep them at their nutritional peak. Caution: Since sprouts are frost sensitive, do not place stored sprouts near the freezer compartment.

SPROUT GARDEN METHOD

This method is just as easy as the jar method. It is also the best way to sprout several kinds of seeds such as beans and grains at the same time. One of the best sprouting trays for this purpose is the Sprout Garden. The bottom of this sprouting tray is covered with holes for good drainage, and will keep even the smallest seed from falling through. The dividers give an advantage over the jar method by allowing you to sprout different seeds separately in each compartment. The depth of the tray and the many holes promote good air circulation. The protective cover keeps out dust, mold spores and insects. Another popular use is to plant an indoor garden with soil (forest mulch). The Sprout Garden is very handy for quickly producing a fine crop of wheatgrass, sunflower, or buckwheat lettuce in just a few days.

There are three pre-mixed salad combinations available from Living Whole Foods distributors. The 3-part salad mix contains alfalfa, broccoli, and radish seed. When sprouted, they "fluff up" together into a delightful, tasty combination. They are good alone, together, or mixed with other salad fixings. The 5-part salad mix contains mung beans and lentils besides the above three. This creates a denser, higher fiber salad. Or this mix can be added to soups for a hearty flavor and nutritional boost. The bean salad contains mung and adzuki beans with lentils and radish seed. Adzuki beans are high in fiber, protein, calcium, iron, vitamins A, B-1, B-2 and niacin. This combination is good by itself, or added to various vegetable dishes. The salad mixes can be sprouted using either the jar or tray method.

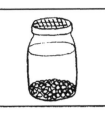

Step One: Start with 2 to 4 table-spoons of small seeds or 4 to 6 table-spoons of large ones. Rinse and then soak in the provided sprouter covers. When sprouting different kinds, use different covers. Be sure to cover to protect from light.

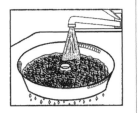

Step Two: Spread the soaked and swollen seeds over the "seed bed" in a tray compartment. Rinse under the faucet gently and allow the seeds to spread evenly.

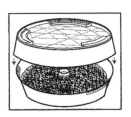

Step Three: Use the cover to protect from light and possible airborne con-taminants. Use the extra sprout cover as a drain board on the bottom and stack all three sprouters if you're using them all. Place the tray in a suitable warm location around 70 degrees.

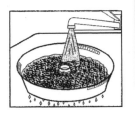

Step Four: Rinse two or three times daily. Check the bottom of the tray for signs of mold. If you find any, wipe it off with a paper towel and rinse again.

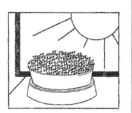

Step Five: In a day or two, tiny leaves will begin to appear on sprouts such as alfalfa, cabbage etc. Uncover any compartment containing these to allow indirect light to enter, but do not place in direct sunlight. Use each cover underneath each sprouter tray as a drain board and pour out any excess drainage each day.

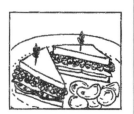

Step Six: Harvest by cleaning to remove hulls and drain well. Hulls may rinse out easily by pouring the water through the exit ports on the side of the trays.

CHIA AND FLAX

Sprouting chia and flax requires some special effort due to their unique qualities. Even though they are a bit more work, the results are well worth the effort. Chia and flax seeds cannot be sprouted using conventional tray or jar sprouters, and must be dry sprouted. There are two different approaches to dry sprouting them, but we recommend the terra-cotta dish approach:

OUR PREFERRED METHOD:
1. Sprinkle a thin layer of chia or flax seed on the bottom of a terra-cotta non-glazed dish or plate.
2. Set the terracotta dish in a larger plate of water.
3. Cover with another plate.
4. Small amounts of water permeate the terra-cotta plate on which the seeds are sitting, and provide exactly the right amount of water to sprout them.
5. On the second day, lightly mist the seeds.
6. Harvest on the third day.
7. It takes about two or three days to get healthy sprouts.

AN ALTERNATE METHOD:

1. Lay a nylon or linen cloth on a plate.
2. Spray a fine mist of water onto the cloth.
3. Sprinkle one layer of chia or flax seed on top of the bag and mist it lightly.
4. Cover with another plate, misting lightly once per day.
5. You will have sprouts in about two to three days.

Sample taste your growing sprouts occasionally to find when they taste best to your palate. If possible, use a carbon filter if your water supply contains chlorine. Space rinsing times evenly over the day. Morning and evening rinsing is usually easiest.

The following chart lists all the sprouting seeds and salad mixes available from the Living Whole Foods. It condenses the basic sprouting information you will need into a simple, handy guide. Happy sprouting!

SPROUTING CHART

SEED	METHOD	AMOUNT QT. JAR	SOAK HOURS	TEMP.	RINSE/ DAY	DAYS	HARVEST INCHES
Alfalfa[1]	Jar/Tray	1½ Tbsp	6–8	65-85	2-3x	4–6	1½–2
Barley	Soil	1-2 Cups	10–12	65-85	2x	7–10	4–8
Bean Salad[1,4]	Jar/Tray	Cup	10–12	65-85	2-3x	2–5	¼–3
Broccoli	Jar/Tray	2 Tbsp	6–8	65-85	2-3x	4–6	1 – 1½
Buckwheat	Soil	1 Cup	10–12	65-80	2-3x	8–15	4½–6
Chinese Cabbage[1]	Jar/Tray	2 Tbsp	6–8	65-85	2-3x	3–5	1 – 1½
Fenugreek[3]	Jar/Soil	¼ Cup	8–12	65-85	2x	3–6	1–2
Garbanzo	Jar/Tray	1 Cup	12	65-85	2--3x	2–3	½–1
Green Pea	Jar/Tray	1 Cup	12	65-85	2-3x	2–3	½
Lentil	Jar/Tray	¾ Cup	8–12	60-85	2-3x	2–4	¼–1
Mung Bean[2]	Jar/Tray	Cup	12–18	70-85	3-4x	3–5	1–3
Radish[1]	Jar/Soi[1]	2 Tbsp	6–8	65-85	2-3x	4–5	1–2
Red Clover[1]	Jar/Tray	2 Tbsp	6–8	65-85	2-3x	4–6	1½–2
Red Winter Wheat	Tray/Soil	1 Cup	10–12	55-75	2x	2–3	¼–½ (grass 6-8)
Soybean	Jar/Tray	½ Cup	12	65-85	2-3x	2–5	½
Sunflower	Tray/Soil	1 Cup	10–14	60-80	2x	2–4	3–5
3-Part Salad Mix[1,4]	Jar/Tray	1½ Tbsp	6–8	65-85	2-3x	2–5	1 – 1½
5-Part Salad Mix[1,4]	Jar/Tray	2 Tbsp	6–8	65-85	2-3x	2–5	¼–3

NOTES:

1. Soak less time during the heat of the summer.
2. Green with light during last day to develop chlorophyll.
3. Grow in dark, allow to soak for a minute when rinsing.
4. Will get bitter if allowed to develop green leaves.
5. Cold final rinse extends storage life.

HOW TO USE SPROUTS

Sprouts are vegetables. They can therefore be used in all vegetable dishes. The easiest, tastiest and most nutritious way to use them is uncooked such as in sprout salads or on sandwiches instead of lettuce. Since vitamins and enzymes are lost in cooking, sprouts should be added during the last stages of cooking. A few sprouts—such as sprouted wheat—can even be used in baking.

MAKING CRACKERS

Allow the wheat sprouts to drain and dry for three to six hours before grinding. Wet sprouts will not grind well and will create too much moisture in the dough. Use a food processor, Champion juicer, wheatgrass juicer or meat grinder. Other juicers or blenders are not designed to grind and should not be used. After grinding, you should end up with a smooth paste. Lumpy, coarse or chunky dough will not work nearly as well, and should be ground a second time. Now you are ready to form the loaves.

After washing your hands to prepare, you have two options. You can oil your hands with a corn, sunflower or sesame seed oil and knead the dough, folding it into itself several times. This will spread the gluten and help the bread stick together and rise better. Or you can go straight to shaping the loaves before popping them in the oven. Just form balls of dough about 3 inches in diameter. You should get two to four loaves from the 2 cups of wheat you began with. Place them on a flat baking tray such as a cookie sheet. You may wish to dust the tray with corn meal or sesame seeds to prevent sticking, Oiling a baking tray is not recommended because heat makes oils indigestible. Now flatten each ball to a height of about 1 ½ inches and a diameter of 4 to 5 inches. For a tastier bread, you may wish to mix your own "additives" into the dough. You can add dates, raisins, chopped nutmeats, nutbutters, coconut, cinnamon, vanilla, etc. for a real taste treat.

NUTRITIONAL GAINS
Sprouting seeds results in the following nutritional improvements:

- Vitamin E content has tripled.

- Starches such as gluten are now simple sugars like maltose.

- Minerals are freed up for easy assimilation.

- Enzymes are plentiful and have converted starches to sugars, proteins to amino acids and fats into essential fatty acids.

- Now contains three to four times more fiber than stone-ground whole wheat bread.

- Thanks to the natural sugars, sprouted wheat bread is sweet as well as nutritious.

Wheat and wheat-based breads are a staple food in the diet of over half the world's population. Unfortunately in the new millennium, many breads on supermarket shelves are not very nutritious. During the milling process the live portion with most of the nutrients—the germ—is removed to prevent spoilage. Along with it goes the wheat bran or fiber that aids elimination. What remains is basically a sticky starch called gluten (also used in wallpaper paste).

To this is added a host of chemical additives which make white bread one of the most chemically-contaminated foodstuffs available today.

SPROUT BREAD

You can't rush a sprout bread. Pre-heat your oven to 250 degrees and place the baking tray with loaves on the center rack. Bake for 2 ½ to 3 ½ hours at 250 degrees depending on the size of the patties and your oven. This low temperature, long-term baking method preserves most of the nutrients from heat. Although the oven temperature may be 250 degrees, the temperature inside the loaves is about 100 degrees cooler. You may wish to use a spatula midway in the baking to lift the bread from the tray to prevent sticking. The bread is ready when the top of each loaf is firm to the touch but not hard. The loaves should still be moist like brownies when removed from the oven,

This delicious sprouted wheat bread is denser, chewier, sweeter and tastier than breads made with flour. This method of using sprouted grains in bread-making goes back to biblical times. Such breads can become a major improvement in you and your family's diets. You will get plenty of protein, while consuming fewer calories and none of the additives commonly found in commercial baked products. You can also use a dehydrator if you have one. Keep the drying temperature under 118 degrees Fahrenheit.

Now consider a completely natural, unadulterated, uncontaminated alternative—sprouted wheat bread. All you will need is 2 cups of red winter wheat. Nothing else. After three days of sprouting, when the sprout is as long as the berry from which it springs the following will occur:

• Vitamin B-12 content has quadrupled to around 54

milligrams per 100 grams (versus just one milligram in white bread).

- Other B vitamins have increased three to twelve times.
- Fewer calories.
- Very little fat and no pesticide residues.
- Fewer processing contaminants or chemical additives.

You will enjoy better digestion because of the enzymes and the fiber will aid regularity. By including sprouted wheat bread in your diet, you will be getting the real staff of life for nutritional support. You may even experience a corresponding boost in energy and health which the living germ of the grain can help bestow.

MANY USES OF SPROUTS

There are as many ways to use sprouts in cooking as there are for any vegetables. The difference here is that you will want to cook the sprouts as little as possible in order to protect their vital nutrients. Following are 30 ways to cook with sprouts. The sprouts listed work well, but try others and use your imagination.

1. Add to tossed salads
2. Use in coleslaw - cabbage, clover, radish
3. Try in potato salad - mung bean, lentil
4. Add to jellied fruit salads - alfalfa, clover
5. Use in oriental stir-fry dishes - mung bean·
6. Blend into fruit shakes or juices - alfalfa, clover
7. Blend with vegetable juices - cabbage, mung bean, lentil
8. Replace celery in sandwich spreads - lentil, radish
9. Grind up and use in sandwich spreads -lentil, radish

10. Mix with soft cheeses for a dip - mung bean, radish

11. Top grilled cheese sandwiches after grilling - alfalfa, clover. Vegans may wish to substitute with soy cheese

12. Stir into soups or stews as they cool- mung bean, lentil

13. Use as a breakfast cereal - wheat only

14. Mix into pancake or waffle batter - buckwheat

15. Add to potato pancakes - alfalfa, clover

16. Add to scrambled eggs - alfalfa, clover, radish. Vegans may wish to scramble tofu and add sprouts

17. Mix into omelets - alfalfa, clover, radish

18. Grind up and mash into potatoes - mung bean, lentil, wheat

19. Combine in rice dishes - fenugreek, lentil, mung bean

20. Mix into fried rice as it cools - lentil, mung bean

21. Stir-fry with other vegetables - alfalfa, clover, radish, mung bean, lentil

22. Mix in spaghetti sauce as it cools - alfalfa, clover

23. Sauté with onions - mung bean, clover, radish

24. Puree with peas or beans - mung bean, lentil

25. Add to baked beans - lentil

26. Steam and serve with margarine - mung bean, lentil

27. Use to garnish a plate - alfalfa, clover, salad mixes

28. Mix into camping foods as you cook them - lentil, mung bean

29. Use in sandwiches instead of lettuce - alfalfa, clover, radish

30. Eat them fresh and uncooked in a sprout salad - salad mixes

SPROUTS AS FOOD STORAGE

Sprouting seeds, beans and grains have been a survival method of all cultures since civilization began. Without saving seed from the previous harvest, how would the next seasons harvest begin? Methods of storing of course have improved and there are many, however, the best methods that we've found are listed below.

STORAGE METHODS

Nitrogen Packed - By far the best known method of storing for long term periods is nitrogen packing. When nitrogen gas is added to a can, jar or bucket and quickly sealed the oxygen is immediately dissipated and therefore can not allow microscopic larvae to generate. Larvae exists in some quantity on most foods of this sort and must not be allowed to breathe, or obtain warmth, moisture or light to generate.

Oxidation is another factor that can occur. Removing oxygen preserves the life force of the item being stored.

Number 10 sealed and nitrogenized cans seem to last the longest with reported shelf life of up to ten years. But more realistically twelve to fifteen years depending on the item stored and storing conditions. It is best to store food-grade nitrogenized cans in a cool dry place for long term periods. (See list of availability of pre-packed nitrogenized seeds and grains or look up web site www.wheatgrasskits. com for more information. We guarantee our seeds for two years!)

Dry Ice - Storing in 5-gallon plastic buckets with dry ice at the bottom and pouring the product on top immediately applying a rubber sealed lid can be used. The nitrogen from the dry ice is emitted and an oxygen reduction factor occurs often times keeping the product bug free for reported periods of up to four or five years. Problems can arise if the plastic buckets become brittle over time and crack or simply breathe air through the plastic thereby defeating the purpose.

Dry ice will also burn sensitive seeds and grains upon contact which will then simply refuse to sprout when the time comes.

NATURAL CONTROLS

Bay Leaves - An old time tested and less expensive method of storing food with bay leaves has been successful as well.

Simply spread four to five bay leaves flat around the storing container and layer the product 4 to 5 inches placing more bay leaves at each layer until container is full. Seal container and check for infestation every few months to be sure. Since there are no gases to escape, food storage can be checked more often. While this is an older method of storage, there are no guarantees in the long run of one day opening up that proverbial can of worms!

Freezing – Freezing seeds has proven to keep seeds viable indefinitely. If you freeze seeds, avoid opening and closing the container you have them in. If you must open the container to remove seed, do not open when the air is particularly humid as it will condense in the container. The drier the air in the container, the better.

Diatomaceous Earth – This can be used to protect seed against insect attack. If larvae or eggs are in the stored seed, when they hatch the dust acts as a desiccant and as a cutting agent, killing the insect as it tries to move about in the container.

CRUCIFEROUS NUTRITION

All members of the cruciferous family of green vegetables, broccoli, kale and spinach, offer a wide range of benefits to biogenic greens. These foods are rich in iron, oxalic acid, chlorophyll, carotenoids, lutein, zeaxanthin, indoles, vitamin A and C and fiber. Broccoli and broccoli sprouts also contain a powerful antioxidant "sulphoraphane" which helps human cells fight the progression of free radicals. A study of researchers at John Hopkins University reveals that broccoli sprouts have up to fifty times more anticancer chemicals in them than in the mature vegetable.

Broccoli sprouts (raw): Provide vitamins A, B, and C; potassium and the phytochemicals sulforaphane; indole and isothiocyanate. Research suggest these phytochemicals may reduce the risk of breast, stomach, and lung cancers.

SERVING SIZE 3oz. (85g) SERVING 1			
AMOUNT PER SERVING			
Calories	35	Calories from Fat 5 %	Daily Value*
Total Fat	0.5g		1%
Saturated Fat	0g 0%	Cholesterol 0mg	0%
Sodium	25mg		1%
Total Carbohydrates	5g 2%	Dietary Fiber 4g	16%
Protein	2g		
Vitamin A			10%
Vitamin C			60%
Calcium			6%
Iron			4%

The following article describes some of the recent findings regarding broccoli sprouts and how they provide nutritional benefits that can help in our ongoing efforts to overcome diseases that seem hopeless.

RECENT STUDY

Study finds broccoli sprouts have high levels of anti-cancer chemical:

Washington (AP) - Good news for people who hate broccoli: A study shows that there is up to 50 more anti-cancer chemical in broccoli sprouts than in the mature vegetable—and the sprout don't taste like broccoli.

Three-day-old broccoli sprouts, which are tender shoots topped with two baby leaves, are loaded with a concentrated form of sulforaphane, a powerful cancer fighter, says researchers at John Hopkins University.

Dr. Paul Talalay, head of a team at Hopkins that discovered sulforaphane five years ago, said he was surprised that the sprouts contained such a high level of the anti-cancer compound.

"If these are developed commercially this could be a really easy way for people to get the benefits of chemoprotection against cancer," said Talalay.

A report on the research was being published Tuesday in the proceedings of the National Academy of Science.

Earlier studies showed that sulforaphane, found in broccoli, cauliflower and some other vegetables, promotes the body to make an enzyme that prevents tumors from forming. A 1994 study indicated that cancer development was reduced by 60 percent to 80 percent in laboratory animals fed sulforaphane extracted from broccoli.

Talalay said that diet studies have shown that eating two pounds of broccoli a week—an unappetizing thought to many people—can provide enough sulforaphane to lower colon cancer risk by half.

But Talalay said that his lab has found that the sulforaphane content in broccoli from a grocery store can vary by a factor of eight or ten and there is no way to identify a vegetable loaded with the compound from one that is not.

"They look the same," he said. "It is impossible to tell a highly protective broccoli from a poorly protective broccoli."

Broccoli sprouts may solve this problem, said Talalay, because the baby plants have a uniformly high level of sulforaphane.

"Because of the high content (of sulforaphane), it is possible to consume far lower quantities of the sprouts and get the same protection," he said.

Broccoli sprouts resemble the alfalfa sprout now common in grocery stores, but they have more flavor, said Talalay. And the broccoli sprouts do not have the sharp tang of mature broccoli that many people, such as former President Bush, find unpleasant.

"They have a far more interesting taste than ordinary sprouts". said Talalay. "You can use them in sandwiches or salads."

Talalay said the broccoli sprouts take just three days to grow from seeds, in contrast to the 55 to 70 days it takes to grow a mature broccoli plant.

Broccoli sprouts are not now grown commercially, but Talalay said that if other researchers confirm the findings of his lab, it could encourage growers to start producing the baby broccoli as a new vegetable for health-conscious shoppers.

"This is an important finding," said Michael Bennett, a professor at the University of Texas, Southwest Medical Center and an expert on diet and cancer. He said diets rich in broccoli and other vegetables have a proven benefit to health but that "the important thing is getting people to eat them."

With the end of the twenty-first century our society has become more concerned with health than ever before in history. Our lives are constantly bombarded with new studies showing the additives in our food, pollution, radiation, or just plain unhealthy living will inevitably give us cancer. As a society we have accepted cancer as a common constant along with death and taxes, however recent medical studies have shown us how to reduce the chances of getting cancer up to 80 percent with daily intakes of sulforaphane. Sulforaphane is a compound that prevents cancer by "assisting the body to create an enzyme that prevents tumors from forming. The test showed sulforaphane from broccoli reduced cancer by 60 to 80 percent." (Life Extension Dec. 1997) Further studies showed that "sulforaphane aided in shrinking tumors already present" (Dr. David G. Williams. Alternatives Jan. 1998).

SULFORAPHANE

Perhaps the most amazing fact about sulforaphane is that it does not concentrate on certain organs or particular cancers. Because it fights cancers on a cellular level it helps all organs against all forms of cancer. Sulforaphane is found in large quantities in broccoli, and increased levels of thirty to fifty times the potency are found in broccoli sprouts, thus making broccoli sprouts among the most potent anticarcinogens in the food arena. Living Whole Foods has been the leader in promoting health through live whole foods and especially sprouts for over two decades. We supply the home sprouter with everything they need to grow sprouts within the sanctuary of their own home.

Our Broccoli Sprouting Seeds are untreated with pesticides, herbicides, fungicides, chemical fertilizers or mercury, making them among the safest and most nutritious in the industry. Our Broccoli Capsules are made from organically grown broccoli sprouts, carefully vacuum dried to preserve their sulforaphane content. Each 250 mg capsule is the equivalent in sulforaphane to 9 ounces of broccoli sprouts. Broccoli Capsules are lab essayed and quality guaranteed.

SOIL AMENDMENTS

AZOMITE™

Your grass will be more beneficial if you add nutrients to your soil. Azomite™ has sixty-seven major and trace elements, so its name means "A to Z of Minerals Including Trace Elements." Typical analysis shows Azomite™ contains every element that's beneficial to plants and animals, and other elements (micro-nutrients) scientists believe essential for health. Azomite™ is a pinkish powder you can add to your soil. (Add ¼ cup of Azomite™ per one tray of wheatgrass. Stir into the soil.) The root system of your grass absorbs the nutrients. You can get Azomite™ from www.wheatgrasskits.com. Or, you can use other organic products to enrich your soil such as earthworm castings, phosphate rock dust, or powdered kelp.

Azomite™ is a natural mined product. For over fifty years regional livestock and crop producers have utilized this unique material from central Utah to improve livestock and plant growth. Assays reveal that the material contains a broad spectrum of metabolically active minerals and trace elements.

Azomite™ is a naturally mined mineral product that requires no mixing. It is odorless, won't burn plants and won't restrict aeration or water penetration. Unlike some products, Azomite™ is not a manufactured, chemically prepared fertilizer. It is 100 percent natural with no additives, synthetics or filters.

Mineralogically, the material can be described as a rhyolitic tuff breccia, which is a hard rock formation formed from the dust of a volcano that exploded, much like when Mount St. Helens did in 1980. Its uniqueness does stem from the multitude of trace minerals found in the deposit. Thus the trade name, Azomite™, means the "A to Z of Minerals Including Trace Elements." Chemically, Azomite™ is a hydrated sodium calcium aluminosilicate (HSCAS) containing other minerals and trace elements which the National Research Council recognizes to be essential. HSCAS is listed in the U.S. Code of Federal Regulations (21 CFR 582.2729) as an anti-caking agent, and is generally recognized as safe (GRAS) by the FDA.

EARTHWORMS AND CASTINGS

Ann Wigmore had a worm bin and let her worms compost all of the used wheatgrass, sunflower, and buckwheat mats. This operation was located right in the basement of the Boston mansion. In all her simplicity, Ann Wigmore had great knowledge about nature and soil and its importance in supplying plants with the correct 'food' for them to build enzyme rich substances that would sustain their life as a healthy plant.

Experiments with worm castings and worms show an increased yield of 20 to 25 percent more grass from the same tray, when 3 tablespoons of castings is added per tray. Edward Howell, famous researcher and nutritionist, had this to say about castings:

In connection with the enrichment of the soil, the enzyme contributions of earthworms should not be ignored. Charles Darwin realized the part worms have played in building soil and wrote a treatise on the subject. In the act of burrowing through the earth, worms engulf the soil, and extract usable materials as food. After passing through the length of the worm, the remainder is expelled in the form of casts which contain a valuable contribution of worm enzyme excretions. The earthworms, like all other animals, continually take in enzymes and eliminate them in their excretions, giving the soil an endowment of free enzymes. Soil rich in worm casts is sought after by some horticulturists for the cultivation of favored plants. It makes high-grade plant food. Worms not only add enzymes to the soil but also loosen it, permitting water and air deeper access. (*Enzyme Nutrition*, by Edward Howell pp.157-159):

We must consume the best quality foods grown from healthy soils. As pointed out, use of castings increased yield up to 25 percent. Dr. Howell points out that the nutritional value of the entire crop is improved if grown in soil where there is significant worm activity. Remember, worm castings are biologically safe and contain no pathogens.

TOXIC BUILD-UP

We can turn for help to another little miracle. A tiny one that we may have overlooked. Consider the parable of the mustard seed. Inside this tiny little seed rests the future mighty plant. A plant that will be many times larger than that tiny germ of life from which it sprouts. A plant that will produce many more seeds, each with another plant resting inside. The mustard seed, then, is much more than a symbol of infinity and of man: it is infinity itself in living form.

Every seed is a plant embryo, waiting for the right conditions to respond with life and germinate into a shooting plant body. Some, like ancient Egyptian wheat, wait for thousands of years. When a seed meets the right combination of moisture, air and temperature, it begins to sprout forth very fast. Just like us, it strives to emerge into the world with a healthy body and to grow up big and strong. For this reason, sprouting seeds produce a wide and abundant array of concentrated vitamins, minerals, trace elements, enzymes, growth hormones, amino acids, simple sugars, <u>essential</u> fatty acids—all of which are essential to human health as well. These nutrients are charged with energy—the energy of life. Instead of nine months, however, these sprouts are ripe and ready for the world in just a few days.

LIVE FOODS

Live foods—of which sprouting seeds, beans and grains are but one category—are beneficial, natural sources of concentrated healthful nutrition. Sprouts can help a body that is constantly exposed to toxic chemicals and is undergoing immune system decline. If we include sprouts in our diets, we give our body the nutrients and energy it needs to cleanse, detoxify, rebuild and heal itself. Then those trillions of tiny cells that make up our comparatively enormous body can continue to do what they do best—keep us alive, alert and feeling healthy.

Annual human adipose (fat) tissue surveys and studies by clinical ecologists are confirming and documenting a steady and alarming build-up of toxic chemical residues in the entire American population. Several of the toxins detected are so dangerous at any level that they have been placed on the EPA "banned" list—a list which keeps getting longer. But banning them—and the thousands of others which have not yet been tested for toxicity—will do nothing about the millions of tons of toxic chemicals that already permeate our environment. They will continue to build up in our bodies, unless we personally take corrective action. No one knows the full consequences of all these different chemicals combining in the human body. Especially when that same body is also exposed to various harmful biological and radiological agents as well. But thanks to widespread contamination of our environment, we are all guinea pigs in a giant experiment resulting from our wasteful and destructive chemical, biological and radiation technologies. If we wish to avoid possible future suffering and ill health, we need to do something about toxic build-up.

SYMPTOMS OF TOXIC BUILDUP

One clinical indication of toxic build-up is chemical allergy. Blood and urine tests of chemically-allergic people invariably reveal high concentrations of various toxic chemical residues in their bodies. The Toxicity Chart lists some of the symptoms of chemical allergy caused by toxic build-up. (page 71)

These symptoms need to be heeded. None of these conditions are normal. If you are experiencing any of them, your body is trying to tell you something. If you already know you are allergic to certain chemicals, you may wish to seek out a physician trained in clinical ecology for testing and treatment. More chemicals, pain-relievers, antihistamines, antacids, etc, - will only make matters worse. They only temporarily relieve or cover-up symptoms, without doing anything about or even aggravating the cause - toxic build-up. Some clinical ecologists estimate that 1 in 10 Americans are already reaching the danger point - toxic overload. At this stage, internal damage leads to organ failure and various health emergencies. Toxic build-up is one of the primary causes of the present runaway epidemics of infectious, contagious and degenerative diseases in the industrialized world, especially in the urban United States. These damaging toxins are also called free radicals.

CHEMICAL ALLERGY FACTORS

Lipid Peroxides. These are fat molecules stripped of electrons and made into free radicals by the two other kinds when they attack lipids, or fats. Free radicals can be very damaging inside the human body. One free radical can destroy an enzyme, even an entire cell. Free radicals cause four basic kinds of physical damage:

1. **Cross-linking.** This is when free-radical damage causes protein, RNA, and DNA molecules—even whole cells—

to fuse together, altering or halting their normal activities. This damage is most visibly evident in the skin, where it causes wrinkling.

2. **Lysosome Destruction.** Lysosomes are cell digestive enzymes. When altered or released into the cell uncontrollably, they can destroy critical cell components, even the entire cell itself. A common symptom of this damage is inflammation, such as that found in arthritis and rheumatism.

3. **Cell Membrane Destruction.** Cell and tissue membranes are composed of lipids (fats) which assist passage of nutrients into cells and wastes out of them. When damaged by free radicals, these fats become insoluble, and the cell wall gradually becomes a "stone wall," This damage eventually leads to cell dysfunction and cell death.

4. **Lipid (Fat) Peroxidation.** Its more common name is rancidity, the end result of fats and oils "going bad." Once cell membranes and fatty tissue begin to go rancid under attack from free-radicals, this creates a cascade of thousands more free radicals. Rancidity is free radical damage that is out of control. It is one of the primary causes of disease in this "chemical age" and can be expected to take an even higher toll throughout the new millennium.

Free-radical damage is a fact of life in the twenty first[t] century. It comes not just from the toxic chemical residues (hydrocarbons, heavy metals, etc), but also from exposure to: environmental radiation (X-rays, microwaves, TV), solar radiation (ultraviolet light), food irradiation, nuclear waste, poor nutrition (especially fried fats and oils), illness (where there is cellular destruction), even emotional stress and distress which is difficult to avoid in many fast-paced and tension-filled lives.

CHEMICAL ALLERGY INDICATORS

Skin: Itching, burning, flushing, tingling, sweating behind neck, hives, blisters, blotches, red spots, chloracne, weals, itchy rashes, psoriasis, dermatitis.

Ear, nose, throat: Nasal congestion, sneezing, nasal itching, runny nose, post-nasal drip. Sore, dry, or tickling throat, clearing throat, itching palate, hoarseness, hacking cough. Fullness, ringing, or popping of ears, earache, intermittent deafness, dizziness, imbalance. Recurrent throat or ear infections.

Eyes: Blurring of vision, pain in eyes, watery eyes, crossing of eyes, glare hurts eyes. Eyelids twitching, drooping or swollen, Redness or swelling of inner angle of lower lid.

Respiratory: Shortness of breath, wheezing, persistent cough, mucus formation in bronchial tubes, recurrent respiratory infections.

Cardiovascular: Pounding heart, increased or racing pulse rate, skipped beats, flushing, pallor, hot flashes, chills or cold extremities, redness or blueness of hands, faintness, chest pain.

Gastrointestinal: Dryness of mouth, increased salivation, canker sores, stinging tongue, burping, retasting, heartburn, indigestion, nausea, vomiting, difficulty in swallowing, rumbling in abdomen, abdominal pain, cramps or colitis, alternating diarrhea and constipation, itching or burning of rectum, food intolerances, bloating, gas, sluggishness after eating.

Nervous system: Headache, migraines, dizziness, light-headedness, compulsively sleepy, drowsy, slower reflexes, depressed; anxious, stimulated, over active, tense, restless, jittery, easily irritated; silly, inebriated, unable to concentrate, trouble remembering words or numbers or names; stammering or stuttering speech, panic attacks and chronic anxiety, delusions or hallucinations, twitching, tremors, convulsions.

FREE RADICAL DAMAGE

Normal molecules have pairs of electrons spinning in their outer shells that balance each other for electrical stability. A free radical is any molecule that has an unpaired outer electron. It is "free" to react "radically" with other molecules and cause cellular damage. There are three major kinds of biologically damaging free radicals:

Oxides, superoxides and hydroxyls both are unbalanced forms of oxygen. Superoxides are oxygen molecules (0^2) lacking an outer electron. Oxides are singlet oxygen atoms (0^2) that lack an electron. Both are highly reactive inside the human body.

Hydroxyls (HO) are an unbalanced, free-radical form of water (H_2O) which lacks the balancing electron of the missing hydrogen atom. This is the most reactive free radical known.

AGING AND HEART DISEASE

Strong body odor is one indication that rancidity is occurring inside the body due to free-radical damage, With the continued build-up of fat in human bodies will come more damage from free radicals because most chemical toxins are fat soluble. This means that they readily combine and react with fatty tissue while building up inside it. Consequently, the more fat and toxic build-up in a person's body, the more cellular damage, ill health, and faster aging there will be in that body.

Toxic build-up can add to the cause of heart disease. Arteriosclerosis, or hardening of the arteries, results from cholesterol (fat) build-up and free-radical attack which hardens it onto the artery walls. This combined with toxic fatty build-up around the heart itself contributes to the ever-increasing incidence of heart disease in this country.

Changing to a raw or mostly raw vegan diet, rich in sprouts and wheatgrass juice, will alleviate all of these problems.

ANTIOXIDANTS

Toxins accumulating in the pelvic areas cause lower immune response, increasing the likelihood of infection and subsequent spread of disease. Toxic residues, therefore, are a major contributing factor in the spread of many diseases. At the same time, several strains are adapting to their toxic environment by developing immunity to various antibiotics (which also contribute to toxic buildup). The increased incidence of cancer in the excretory and reproductive organs may also be partly attributable to this toxic build-up.

NATURE'S PROTECTORS

Our body's first and primary line of defense against free-radical (oxidant) attack are the antioxidants supplied in our diet. These natural substances neutralize free radicals by combining with them chemically to render them harmless. They go even further, and are vital in nourishing, strengthening and stimulating the immune system. Some antioxidants are vitamins, others are minerals or trace elements, still others are enzymes and plant pigments. All of them, to one degree or another, can protect us from toxic chemical build-up and attack. Let's take a closer look at the twelve most important ones, all of which occur abundantly in various sprouting seeds, beans, and grains.

VITAMINS

Provitamin A (Carotenes) - This is by far one of the best antioxidants and immune system builder. The synthetic form of vitamin A (another chemical) is toxic to the body in large doses. When derived from carotenes (provitamin A) it is completely nontoxic. Our body merely stores any excess in the liver and fatty tissue, Since this is where most toxic residues also get stored, provitamin A can help keep fatty tissue from becoming rancid. Vitamin A is essential in the diet for healthy epithelial tissue. This tissue forms the skin, glands such as the mammary glands and the mucous membranes which line the lungs and the digestive, urinary and intestinal tracts. Vitamin A deficiency has been linked with higher incidence of cancer in epithelial tissue, which accounts for well over half of all cancers. Optimum dietary levels of vitamin A are known to boost the immune system. Studies have found increased production of lymphocytes, phagocytes, T cells, B cells, and five classes of antibodies, including interferon and tumor necrosis factor. Vitamin A also helps protect the body from radiation, especially solar radiation effects on the skin. With rising levels of ultraviolet radiation falling on us due to a weakened ozone layer, this protection becomes doubly important. Unfortunately, however, according to several studies by the USDA and others, over 50 percent of all American diets are dangerously deficient in this important vitamin and antioxidant. Provitamin A rises dramatically when sprouting seeds that develop chlorophyll are exposed to a few hours of direct sunlight. Sunlight triggers the production of carotenes as well.

Vitamin B Complex - The B Complex includes B-1 (thiamine), B-2 (riboflavin), B-3 (niacin), B-6 (pyridoxine), B-12 (cyanocobalamin), B-13 (orotic acid), B-15 (pangamic acid), B-17 (laetrile), folic acid, pantothenic acid, biotin, inositol, choline, and PABA. The B vitamins aid in the metabolism of proteins and fats, boost energy and help the immune system produce antibodies. They also help regulate the important elimination organs of the liver and kidneys. One of the highest natural sources of B vitamins is sprouted grains.

Toxic chemical residues tend to accumulate and concentrate in the pelvic areas for two major reasons. First, this area is where most people carry a large portion of their body fat. As we learned earlier, toxins tend to lodge in fatty tissue. Second, this is also where the excretory organs are located. Toxins that cannot be excreted tend to linger in and migrate into the reproductive organs, where they can damage sperm and ova—even DNA, the "genetic blueprint" for future generations.

Although we can't escape these toxic poisons completely, we can do something to slow, stop or even reverse toxic build-up. Obviously, the more we expose our body to toxic chemicals, the more toxic our body will become. The first step, then, is to slow toxic build-up by decreasing our toxic intake. This means watching what we eat, drink, breathe and allow our skin to come in contact with. This also means decreasing our intake of saturated fats, especially fried foods or fats and oils cooked at high temperatures, stored for a long time, or overly exposed to air and light. To stop or reverse toxic build-up, we will need to go further and increase our toxic output, This means adding nutrients in our diet known to neutralize these poisons and help our body eliminate them. This is where sprouts come in. They contain all the nutrients needed in a delicious and readily available form.

Vitamin C - This important vitamin directly neutralizes and detoxifies over fifty known chemical toxins. For example, it keeps cancer-causing chemicals known as nitrosamines from forming from nitrates. Vitamin C also boosts the immune system. It increases the production of disease-fighting lymphocytes and the production of interferon. It increases iron assimilation and helps prevent anemia. Fresh-squeezed citrus juices are one good source, but some sprouts and sprout juices are even higher in vitamin C content.

Vitamin E - This vitamin provides a host of antioxidant qualities. It prevents rancidity of fats in the bloodstream and elsewhere in the body, especially the skin. It also protects enzymes, hormones and other antioxidants. Vitamin E boosts the oxygen-carrying capacity of red blood cells and helps oxygenate body tissues. It strengthens the immune system and assists production of T cells, B cells, and several antibodies. Cold-pressed wheat germ oil is one way to add it to your diet. However sprouted wheat, alfalfa, or clover cost much less.

Chlorophyll - Although it is neither a vitamin nor a mineral, chlorophyll is a potent antioxidant and blood purifier. It has been called "green blood," and for good reason. Its molecular structure is identical to that of the heme molecule in red blood cells, except it has magnesium instead of iron at the center. Since our body converts chlorophyll to heme in producing new red blood cells, it is essential in the diet for a healthy, oxygen-rich blood supply. Unfortunately, many American diets are deficient in this important antioxidant.

Chlorophyll is known to fight infections by retarding the growth of bacteria, especially odor-causing bacteria. For this reason, it is not just a great detoxifier, but a natural deodorizer as well. In combination with calcium phosphate found in sprouted grains, it helps neutralize fluorides that may enter the body via the water supply. Chlorophyll also stimulates tissue cell activity and its normal regrowth. It is therefore essential in the diet for rebuilding blood and tissues damaged by toxic chemicals.

The highest levels of chlorophyll, up to 70 percent of solid's content, are found in cereal grasses such as wheatgrass after they are juiced and strained. Wheatgrass juice provides many other important antioxidant vitamins, minerals and enzymes for quick assimilation into the bloodstream. For this reason, a later section will explain how to grow and juice wheatgrass. Wheatgrass juice is also the best source for the antioxidant enzymes discussed below.

Vitamins and chlorophyll remove free radicals directly. The following minerals and trace elements work indirectly by activating the antioxidant enzymes which will be covered later.

MINERALS

Calcium - Calcium helps the kidneys eliminate toxins. It helps regulate blood pH and electrolyte balance. Calcium helps the body eliminate heavy metals such as cadmium, lead and mercury, and radioactive isotopes such as Strontium 90.

Iron - This mineral, found in every cell in the body, is essential in the production of hemoglobin, the oxygen-carrying component in red blood cells. Iron also improves immune response by strengthening respiratory action and tissue oxygenation. It has been found to prevent absorption of heavy metals such as lead and cadmium.

Magnesium - This important mineral, a component of chlorophyll, has many protective functions in the body. It helps counteract aluminum toxicity, balances the properties of calcium, and aids in the utilization of many other antioxidants by the body. The RDA for magnesium is 350 milligrams, which is easily supplied by a diet which includes chlorophyll-rich sprouts.

Potassium - This helps maintain normal mineral balance and effective mineral function. It helps detoxify the kidneys. It also prevents over acidity by maintaining the acid-alkaline balance in the blood and tissue. Sprouted wheat and sunflower seeds are good sources of potassium.

Selenium - This trace element is known to fortify and strengthen the immune system by boosting antibody production. It helps the body to attack free radicals, especially hydrocarbons and heavy metals such as lead and mercury. Agriculture chemicals, acid rain and food processing all destroy selenium and all the other antioxidants.

Zinc - This trace mineral is essential to the thymus gland in the production of virus-killing T cells. Zinc is required in the production of nucleic acids such as RNA and DNA, which also help protect against toxic attack. It is also important in the proper absorption and functions of several antioxidant vitamins, especially the B complex. Food processing destroys zinc, especially in the milling of whole grains into refined flour products.

Antioxidant Enzymes - This is a group of metabolic catalysts used by the body specifically to rid itself of free radicals. These are the "activators" of the free-radical disposal system. They include two primary members, superoxide dismutase (SOD) and catalase (CAT), and eight secondary members, including glutathione perioxidase (GP) and methionine reductase (MR).

Each is known to neutralize or deactivate a certain kind of free radical. And where it takes one molecule of a vitamin to neutralize one free radical, a single molecule of one of these enzymes can get rid of thousands. SOD eradicates the superoxides and oxides. GP takes care of the very dangerous lipid peroxides. And MR eliminates the hydroxyls. CAT neutralizes the hydroxyls and assists the others in reducing all the free radicals to harmless end products that the body can then more easily expel. All are found in sprouts, especially in sprouted wheat.

Your body's ability to digest and absorb nutrients from the food you eat is totally dependent on enzymes. Digestion is an enzymatic process from beginning to end. Yet enzyme activity in the average person declines by 30 percent to 50 percent by middle age. This is not surprising when we look at what destroys enzymes. Cooking any food above 140 degrees F destroys them, as does pasteurization.

Food processing destroys enzymes, as well as chlorine and fluoride in drinking water, lead, cadmium and hydrocarbons in air, depressants such as alcohol, stimulants such as caffeine and nicotine, and antibiotics and other drugs. Dietary enzyme deficiency may be a primary cause of digestive disorders and nutrient malnutrition. You can get enzyme sufficiency in your life by adding some sprouts to your diet.

SELECTED ARTICLES

A SHORT HISTORY OF WHEATGRASS AND BARLEY GRASS
by KK Fowlkes

Wheatgrass juice is very sweet tasting, while barley grass juice is mildly bitter. In fact neither grass made into juice tastes very good–but they do deliver improved health.

Interesting: The first recorded mention of a 'grass cure' is found in the Old Testament, Book of Daniel 4:31-32. Grass is apparently recommended as a treatment for Nebuchadnezzar's madness.

> 31. While the word was in the king's mouth, there fell a voice from heaven, saying, O king Nebuchadnezzar, to thee it is spoken; the kingdom is departed from thee.

> 32. And they shall drive thee from men, and thy dwelling shall be with the beasts of the field: they shall make thee to eat grass as oxen, and seven times shall pass over thee, until thou know that the most High ruleth in the kingdom of men, and giveth it to whomsoever he will.

During the early 1900s a man named Edmund Bordeaux Szekely discovered an ancient biblical manuscript, which he subsequently translated. It was a remarkable discovery and Szekely was so enthralled with the translation that he formed a society he called the Biogenic Society to promulgate the teaching of this ancient way of eating. He began publishing the manuscripts in the form of booklets, which he sold inexpensively because he felt that the world needed the message. He called the books "The Essene Gospel of Peace." The Essenes were a righteous people who lived near the Dead Sea during the time of Jesus Christ. According to the "Essene Gospel of Peace" Christ actually taught them the laws of health during that time. The main teaching of Essene Book I is: Don't kill your food by cooking it. The main teaching of Essene Book IV is: all grasses are good for man and wheatgrass is the perfect food for man. These Essene Booklets can typically be purchased at any health food store.

"In 1930, Charles F. Schnabel started feeding his family grass. Before anyone else, he initiated the movement for the human consumption of grass and devoted his entire life to promoting its nutritional and health benefits. He also succeeded in creating a demand for grass as a premium livestock feed and furthered its role as a profitable and ecological crop for American farmers. His dream was to see grass included as a valuable supplement in the American diet. He knew from his experiments with animals and his research in the laboratory that it boosts nutrition, builds good blood and strengthens immunity. His vision was of an America that would donate grass to feed the hungry worldwide and teach malnourished countries to grow it. He is a forgotten hero, but he is remembered for how close he came to making wheatgrass a household food. Few people are aware of it today, but in the 1940s, pharmacies all over America and Canada sold "tins" of grass. Stories about the human consumption of grass appeared in *Newsweek, Business Week*, Time and other magazines. Today, grass is just now approaching the level of popularity that Charles Schnabel had crusaded for and achieved over sixty years ago." (*Wheatgrass, Natures' Finest Medicine,* by Steve Meyerowitz.)

In the 1940s a man by the name of Charles Kettering (former Chairman of the Board of General Motors) donated money for the study of chlorophyll. Chlorophyll was studied intensively by medical doctors using FDA required standards i.e. double blind studies, etc. (There are currently over forty articles written up in medical journals about the healing effects of chlorophyll.) These medical doctors found that chlorophyll was a great healer and used it as such for quite some time. The next question is…why aren't they still using it? Probably because it is hard for anyone to turn a profit on a product like chlorophyll which can be grown in any kitchen or back yard.

Sometime during the 1940s a lady by the name of Ann Wigmore healed herself of cancer from the weeds she found in vacant lots in Boston. (See *Why Suffer* by Ann Wigmore.) She began a study of natural healing modalities–and with the help of a friend, Dr. Earp Thomas, she found that there are 4,700 varieties of grass in the world and all are good for man. (Since that time many more varieties have been discovered.) With the help of her pets, she arrived at the conclusion that wheatgrass was the best medicinal grass. She started an institute in Boston called the Ann Wigmore Institute and since then has taught people from all over the world about the grasses and the living food healing program–and helped them get well from some very serious diseases. She has written over thirty-five books telling about wheatgrass and living foods.

Now, many people are finding out for themselves the great benefits of wheatgrass (which is essentially liquid chlorophyll). Since Ann Wigmore's time, a Japanese researcher named Yoshihide Hagiwara has done research on the healing properties of barley grass. Hagiwara was the owner of a large pharmaceutical company in Japan. He had personally developed numerous medications. He became extremely ill from working with drugs. He came to the conclusion that if synthetic drugs make a person sick, then how could they make one well?

He began to study Chinese medicine and found that the father of Chinese medicine said, "It is the diet which maintains true health and becomes the best drug." Hippocrates, considered the father of western medicine, said basically the same thing. Ann Wigmore originally named her institute after Hippocrates--based on his teaching that the body can act as its own physician when provided with the proper tools (living organic nourishment), used in the way nature intended--unprocessed and uncooked.

Of all the grasses, barley grass has probably been researched more, due to the efforts of Dr. Yoshihide Hagiwara, President of the Hagiwara Institute of Health in Japan. Hagiwara reports that he researched over 150 different plants over a period of thirteen years. He found that in barley was the most excellent source of nutrients that the body needs for growth, repair and well-being.

A biologist named Yasuo Hotta from the University of California, La Jolla, found in barley grass a substance called P4D1. This substance not only has strong anti-inflammatory action but also was shown to actually repair the DNA in the cells of the body. This aided in the prevention of carcinogenesis, aging, and cell death. He reported in a Japan Pharmacy Science Association meeting that P4D1 suppresses or cures pancreatitis, stomatitis, inflammation of the oral cavity, and dermatitis, and also lacerations of the stomach and duodenum. He found that barley juice is much stronger than steroid drugs but has few if any side effects.

Dr. Howard Lutz, who is director of the Institute of Preventive Medicine in Washington, D.C., has said this about barley grass: "[Barley grass is] one of the most incredible products of this decade. It improves stamina, sexual energy, clarity of thought, and reduces addiction to things that are bad for you. It also improves the texture of the skin, and heals the dryness associated with aging."

Some people who first try grass juice find that they have difficulty with wheatgrass juice. It is extremely detoxifying and makes some people nauseous every time they drink it. These people may find that they can much more easily tolerate barley grass juice. It is milder, although bitter, compared to the sweetness of wheatgrass juice. Often barley grass is a good first step to assimilating wheatgrass juice. Barley grass is very high in organic sodium. People who have a tendency towards dehydration need more organic sodium. People with arthritis have used celery juice for years because of the organic sodium it contains. According to Hagiwara, in his book, *Green Barley Essence*, barley grass has 775 mg of organic sodium per 100 grams. This contrasts with 28 mg of sodium per 100 grams in celery. Organic sodium keeps calcium in solution in the bloodstream and also dissolves calcium deposited on the joints. It also replenishes organic sodium in the lining of the stomach. This aids digestion by improving the production of hydrochloric acid in the stomach.

Besides chlorophyll and a myriad of vitamins, minerals and enzymes, barley grass is said to have 30 times as much vitamin B1 as in milk, 3.3 times as much vitamin C, and 6.5 times as much carotene as in spinach, 11 times the amount of calcium in cow's milk, nearly 5 times the iron content of spinach, nearly 7 times the vitamin C in oranges, 4 times the vitamin B1 in whole wheat flour, and 80 micrograms of vitamin B12 per 100 grams of dried barley plant juice. The Resource Research Association, Office of Science and Technology, and Japan Food Analysis Center did this analysis.

This same food analysis center which did research on the dried barley grass juice, found that it contains per 100 grams: 775 organic sodium (natrum), 8,800 potassium, 1,108 calcium, 224.7 magnesium, 15.8 iron, 1.36 copper, 534 phosphorus, 7.33 zinc. Closest to it is spinach: 25 organic sodium (natrum), 490 potassium, 98 calcium, 59.2 magnesium, 3.3 iron, 0.26 copper, 52 phosphorus.

Many people have claimed that regular supplementation with green barley juice stimulates weight loss, which research says is due to the enhancement of the cytochrome oxidase enzyme system which is essential for cell metabolism. Another enzyme contained by barley grass is superoxide dismutase (SOD), a powerful antioxidant which protects the cells against toxic free radicals which are thought to be a primary culprit in aging and many other diseases.

"It has been my experience, after growing both wheatgrass and barley grass and providing juice for people, both in my green house and in juice bars, that people who tend to be arthritic do better with barley grass juice because of its high sodium content. Many people using it have found relief from pain within a week or two. I have also found that people with digestive problems do better with barley grass."

We have Ann Wigmore to thank for her research on wheatgrass and Yoshihide Hagiwara to thank for our knowledge about barley grass. In addition Hippocrates, the father of medicine, advised, "Let your food be your medicine," and Shin Huange-ti said "It is the diet which maintains true health and becomes the best drug."

BARLEY GRASS, THE RESTORER OF HEALTH

by KK Fowlkes

Barley grass, the other green grass! Many people have turned to us to find out why they should try barley grass juice as opposed to wheatgrass. We hope to answer this question. While much of the hype and interest is about wheatgrass; much of the research done on grass was done on barley!

In order to understand the part that barley grass plays in the restoration of health, we must first discuss tentative causes of disease. Let us begin by thinking about the center or the hub of the human body. It is the stomach and the first guardian of the inner sanctum of the body. It is represented around the pupil of the eye and looks much like the hub on a wheel. When the stomach is healthy, the hub is the same color of the iris. When it is unhealthy or deficient in organic sodium it is either lighter or darker than the iris. Lighter is acute, and darker is chronic. We know that the human body is not only physical, mental and spiritual, but is also chemical. It is in the chemical realm where the physical problems of the human body begin.

When a person eats a high animal protein, high sugar and low fiber diet, certain chemical reactions take place in the stomach. A high protein animal diet requires first that the stomach secrete a large amount of hydrochloric acid so that the food can be broken down into amino acids which can be used by the body. In the process of this initial digestion there is always either an acid residue or an alkaline residue. These foods leave an acid residue after the breakdown. This, chyme or food along with the hydrochloric acid that mixes with it in the stomach cannot be allowed to traverse the small and then large intestine as it would do damage to delicate tissues, so the body uses minerals, the chief one being organic sodium, to buffer this acid residue. The lining of the stomach has the greatest amount of sodium in the body and protects the stomach from the hydrochloric acid. The bile that comes from the liver is rich in sodium. This joins with the contents of the stomach to buffer the acid as it leaves the stomach and traverses the intestines.

Day after day, month after month, year after year, if a person eats predominantly the typical American food diet (predominantly flesh foods) which leaves a residue of acid and neglects to eat a high amount of fruits and vegetables which leave an alkaline residue rich in minerals, these minerals, mainly organic sodium, then potassium, then calcium and magnesium are used up.

Dr. Bernard Jensen, known as the father of Iridology, devoted his life to studying and developing iris analysis. Each part of the body and each organ including the brain is represented in the iris of the eye. Each part can look different depending upon the health of the body. Jensen studied and related how the iris changes not only in color but in configuration when certain dietary changes are made. His work contains the basic knowledge of how diet affects the inner tissues and organs of the body. Most importantly he presents his knowledge in before and after pictures so that almost any student can understand the concepts. His work includes the use of foods and certain herbs that are rich in specific minerals to restore health and vitality to different organs or tissues of the body. His many books are used as textbooks for those who wish to learn this fascinating science. It is alternative medicine and is being accepted each year by more and more medical doctors as they eschew drugs and embrace natural medicine. (See *Iridology, the Science and Practice in the Healing Arts. Volumes I and II* by Bernard Jensen, D.C., N.D.)

There are myriads of techniques for drugging or performing surgery upon the human body. Modern allopathic medicine is a method of suppressing the illness. For example if one has a continuous rash, steroids such as cortisone are given to suppress it. The cream pushes the rash or illness further down into the body so that the skin stops breaking out. However, the sickness is still in the body, just further down in the tissues.

Natural medicine seeks to strengthen the tissues using certain foods and plants that are high in organic minerals. When the tissues are strengthened, the body then has the ability to expel the poison or corruption through the skin or wherever it is the easiest. There is no technique that can surpass Jensen's method, because he can actually look into the human body and access information which can be had in no other way and then prescribe those certain foods or herbs which will provide the life giving and healing elements which nourish the tissue of the body, allowing it to strengthen, and then heal itself.

Rich Anderson, student of Dr. Bernard Jensen, and author of Cleanse and Purify Thyself, Volumes I and II says,

When the body becomes low in organic sodium, it is forced to go to another part of its self to retrieve the electrolyte, and it will do this even if it has to kill its own cells. When it begins to retrieve organic sodium from within itself, the most benign and efficient pathway is the bile. This way it can avoid having to directly injure itself. However, the removal of sodium from bile, though harmless in the beginning, has a devastating chain reaction.

The removal of sodium from bile causes the bile pH to drop. The more it drops the more acid it becomes. When bile drops to a certain point, gallstones are formed. Gallstones can cause severe problems, including life-threatening afflictions.

When the bile becomes acid, it is highly caustic and irritates the intestinal wall. Bile can become so acid that it can burn a hole right through the gut wall: In fact 90 percent of all so-called stomach or peptic ulcers are found in the duodenum near the bile duct. Bile irritation is associated with development of polyps, bowl tumors, colon cancer, irritable bowel syndrome (IBS), leaky gut syndrome, and various other bowel diseases.

Fortunately the body has a protective mechanism that can help to compensate for this dangerous scenario: Mucin secretion. Mucin is a glycoprotein mucus. It is secreted by intestinal glands and can line the intestines, thereby protecting it from acids and other irritants. Mucin is the primal essence of mucoid plaque." (Dr. Rich Anderson, Cleanse and Purify Thyself, Volume I)

The good thing about this scenario is that the delicate tissues are protected. The bad part: If the diet stays the same (high animal protein) the mucin continues to form, day after day, year after year, until it has formed a very heavy mucoid plaque which begins to be a home for all kinds of parasites such as harmful bacteria and viruses which were let in by the stomach because a lack of hydrochloric acid couldn't kill them.

The consequences of acid bile and mucoid plaque include the following: poor digestion, poor assimilation, toxic accumulation, poor peristalsis, mutation or destruction of friendly bacteria, bowel diseases, and the commencement of many chronic and degenerative diseases. And all this caused primarily because of organic electrolyte deficiencies or chiefly organic sodium deficiency, because the minerals which are not replaced in the diet become less and less thus exacerbating the problem even further.

The next most likely locale for the body to retrieve organic sodium is the stomach. In a healthy person, the parietal cells of the stomach manufacture hydrochloric acid, an essential element in digestion. But in order to do this, it must have large amounts of organic sodium to protect the stomach cells from the hydrochloric acid. It is at this site that we find the greatest store of organic sodium, and if it is diminished, the stomach is forced to stop hydrochloric acid production. For if the hydrochloric acid production were continued without the protection of organic sodium, the hydrochloric acid would burn a hole right through the stomach. Yes, a lack of organic sodium is associated with ulcers. Therefore, a lack of sodium in the stomach not only means a shutdown of hydrochloric acid production; it also means that pepsinogen cannot be activated, nor can proteins be efficiently digested.

Lack of hydrochloric acid and enzymes devastates digestion. Poor digestion always means that health is diminishing. Not only has that happened, but a lack of the normal hydrochloric acid in the stomach allows potential pathogenic bacteria, parasites, and yeasts to enter the inner sanctum of the gastrointestinal tract." (Dr. Rich Anderson, *Cleanse and Purify Thyself, Volume I*)

Now that the mucoid plaque has become a home for parasites such as harmful fungi, bacteria and viruses other problems arise. One problem is the waste they continually give off, in the process of metabolism and catabolism. This waste in and of itself causes a darkness in the body that is not only physical and chemical but mental. The mucoid plaque prevents our foods from absorbing into the bloodstream properly. Now the cells of our bodies are not only underfed and becoming weaker each day but are surrounded by a murky filth which is hard to cleanse because of the daily inundations of more unhealthy foods.

As the digestive process uses up the organic sodium in the stomach, it then begins to rob it from other parts of the body. If the muscles are robbed, then they become weak. If the joints are robbed of organic sodium, then arthritis begins to develop. Lack of minerals and organic sodium is the beginning of old age as we know it.

What is the good news of this scenario? The good news is that barley grass exists. Barley grass is one of the foods which is extremely high in organic sodium. It contains not only organic sodium but the cleanser chlorophyll. Abstaining from the typical American diet and adding lots of grains, fresh fruits and vegetables along with barley grass juice will begin to restore organic sodium to the stomach and other tissues and the restoration of the health of the human body. Other methods of cleansing the mucoid plaque are found in Rich Anderson's books.

THIS IS HERING'S LAW OF CURE

Constantine Hering, M.D. (1800-1880) observed that healing occurs in a consistent pattern. He described this pattern in the form of three basic laws which homeopaths can use to recognize that healing is occurring. This pattern has been recognized by acupuncturists for hundreds of years and is also used by practitioners of herbalism and other healing disciplines.

According to the first of Hering's laws, healing progresses from the deepest part of the organism—the mental and emotional levels and the vital organs—to the external parts, such as skin and extremities.

Hering's second law states that, as healing progresses, symptoms appear and disappear in the reverse of their original chronological order of appearance. Homeopaths have consistently observed that their patients re-experience symptoms from past conditions.

According to Hering's third law, healing progresses from the upper to the lower parts of the body. For instance, a person is considered to be on the mend if the arthritic pain in his neck has decreased although he now has pain in his finger joints.

As the symptoms change in accordance with Hering's Law, it is common for individual symptoms to become worse than they had been before treatment. If healing is truly in progress, the patient feels stronger and generally better in spite of the aggravation. Before long, the symptoms of the aggravation pass, and leave the person healthier on all levels." (homeoint.org)

Ann Wigmore proved this when in 1950, she began a wellness institute in Boston which remained functional until 1994. There she took people from all over the world and fed them what she called a living food diet. The diet was grown entirely at her institute. There she sprouted many different seeds, buckwheat, alfalfa, sunflower, peas, beans, lentils, etc. and especially wheat which she grew to 6 inches, and harvested and served as wheatgrass juice in addition to the diet of sprouted foods and some organic fruit for taste. Many of the people who went there were in extremely poor health, on their last legs so to speak. They had tried chemotherapy and/or radiation and other traditional forms of medicine, and in a last hope went to Ann. With Ann, they not only regained their health, but their hope. The treatment at the institute lasted for two weeks but the diet was to be followed at least eighteen months. Many people who went on the diet elected to live on it the rest of their lives as they found a palate for this type of food and began to relish the freshness of it and the energy that it created.

The implication that this diet has for all mankind is miraculous. There is a substance in the grasses (wheat, barley) called P4D1 that has been recently discovered by scientists studying barley grass that actually restores and normalizes the genes. With the normalization and the restoration that this diet creates, the world can rid itself of pain, suffering, and children born with genetic problems. Imagine a world with perfect babies. Imagine a world with no tears, no pain, and no sorrows. This is the promise of the millennium, when the lion will lay down with the lamb—when death for all creatures will cease. Health and compassion will reign.

The grasses are a gift from a Creator who foresaw the deterioration of the human race in the last days. It is truly a natural medicine that restores the health and well being of the colonies of organisms that comprise the human body. The body is redeemable. The organisms that comprise it want to live together in harmony and peace. If they are cared for and nourished properly they will change and rejuvenate. They can set the example for the entire race of humans. When the war ends internally, the wars will end externally. Those colonies of organisms (man) when in comfort and peace will only desire to live in comfort and peace with their fellow beings.

DOES THE BODY HAVE THE ABILITY TO HEAL ITSELF?

by KK Fowlkes

In 1822 there was a medical doctor by the name of Isaac Jennings. After 20 years of practicing medicine, he became convinced that drugging and bleeding people did more harm than good. He decided to administer placebos of bread pills, starch powders and colored water to his patients and at the same time instructed them in healthful living habits. By 1822 his fame extended far and wide because of his remarkable healing record. When he finally became convinced that his what he called "The Do-Nothing Cure" worked, he announced his discovery to the world. His announcement was not well received by other doctors or even some of his cured patients who denounced him as an imposter and accused him of cheating them into good health. He continued his practice for another 20 years and helped many people get well.

Current scientists are finding out more and more that what we eat is directly associated with how healthy we are and how we are able to resist sickness and disease through our immune systems. Some of the newest statistics found in recent studies about the differences between vegetarian and non-vegetarian people show some astonishing results. "Some research done by the New England Medical Center and Illinois University School of Medicine show that the chance of obesity, lung cancer, breast cancer and colon diseases are reduced by 40 percent in true vegetarians (vegan) compared to those who are not. Another discovery is that the average man that eats meat has a 50 percent chance of dying from a heart attack while any true vegetarian (vegan) runs only a 4 percent chance.

Also, according to findings that are in the Surgeon General's report on deaths caused by coronary heart disease, we see that there is a definite relationship to those deaths and to their diets. A study of 20,044 vegetarians shows that the rate of mortality, caused by coronary heart disease, among those 35 to 44 years. is 72 percent lower than rates found in the general population. Also the risk of suffering symptoms of coronary heart disease in non-vegetarian males aged 35 to 64 is three times greater than in vegetarian males.

Of the following diseases compared to predominantly vegetarian nations, we (in the US) tend to suffer mostly from arthritis, breast cancer, colon cancer, diabetes, gallstones, heart disease, hyper tension, hypo or hyperglycemia, obesity, prostate cancer, strokes, and others. Now some argue and ask, "Aren't vegetarians undernourished?" The fact is there has not been any evidence that proves that a true vegetarian diet has any bad effects on the body. On the contrary it proves just the opposite: there are only good effects. And this is being proved more and more as research continues. Vegetarianism is regarded by many medical experts to be the ideal form of sustaining good health. And the American Dietetic Association has indicated that one can get all the nutrients they need from a well rounded vegetarian diet. (TL Rodgers, Lifesave.org) When we talk about vegetarian in this article, we are talking about pure vegetarianism, which some people now call vegan.

What are some simple healthful living habits we can adopt in our own lives to maintain or begin to restore our health?

1. Eliminate as much as possible, processed foods (white sugar, white flour, high fat foods, animal protein) from our diet.

2. Gradually go in the direction of eating as much raw or living food as possible: fresh produce, sprouted nuts, grains and seeds, fresh juices, fresh juice of grasses such as barley and wheat.

3. Educate ourselves and our children about our bodies and natural healthful living.

4. Being healthy is really a very simple thing when we go back to nature—not the complicated 10,000 hard to pronounce diseases that ones' medical specialist would have him believe.

5. Be patient. If it took fifteen to thirty years for your body to get into the shape it is in, it might take two or three years of healthful living to get it back into a high state of health. Healthful living builds new tissue to replace the old. It is not a quick fix like a drug.

6. Exercise is very important in that it circulates nutrients to the tissues.

7. Add the grasses to the diet.

8. One hopes that the organic grasses and organic produce such as the greens, have the tiny micro-organ-
   isms that make B-12. If doubtful, it might be well to
   take a B-12 sub-lingual supplement.

If in fact the body does have the ability to heal itself, it
seems that it will do a better job if it is not lugged down
by foods that take hours to digest. Digestion is a major energy drain on the body—energy that could be used to heal
and repair tissue rather than just process food. This is a
major reason that the juices are so effective in their ability
to heal and cleanse. Fresh juice takes about twenty minutes to digest and enter the bloodstream whereas heavy
fat laden destructive type food sometimes takes eight to
twelve hours to be processed before it can be used as
energy for the body. A healthful diet begins when we use
predominantly foods in their natural state.

DETOXIFICATION. . .THE WORD FOR THE DAY

by KK Fowlkes

Detoxification seems to be the word for the day. Never at
a time in the history of man have the foods we eat been
so processed and devitalized. Never has there been the
chemical pollution in the growing soils, in the ground water, the rivers and the oceans and in the air. The shampoos,
lotions, creams, and emollients we slather upon our bodies
have chemical names we've never heard of. Never before
have people suffered en masse from such a wide variety of
illnesses and disease. It is reported that of the 60 million
people who search the internet every day, 20 million are
searching for something to do to improve their health and
immune systems.

In a study led by Mount Sinai School of Medicine in New
York, in collaboration with the Environmental Working

Group and Commonweal, researchers at two major laboratories found an average of 91 industrial compounds, pollutants, and other chemicals in the blood and urine of nine volunteers (one of which was Bill Moyers) with a total of 167 chemicals found in the group. Like most of us, the people tested do not work with chemicals on the job and do not live near an industrial facility. "Scientists refer to this contamination as a person's body burden. Of the 167 chemicals found, 76 cause cancer in humans or animals, 94 are toxic to the brain and nervous system, and 79 cause birth defects or abnormal development. The dangers of exposure to these chemicals-in-combination have not been studied." One can access the website at http://www.ewg.org/reports/bodyburden/es.php

Does body burden equal lethargy or laziness? It is good to know that no one is truly lazy! Body chemistry keeps many people in life from being super-successful. Body chemistry contributes to lethargy, slow mentality, chronic fatigue, disease, old age, and eventually death. So what does it mean to detoxify? Literally it means to clean house. Enabling the body to cleanse itself of toxins means to vitalize the cells of the body so that each cell will have enough energy to empty the garbage so to speak. In other words to rid itself of toxins and in so doing, changing the environment or the body chemistry.

Why don't the cells of our bodies have energy to rid themselves of toxins? As Ann Wigmore has said, and many before her: a devitalized lifeless cooked food diet. Arnold Ehret (Mucusless Diet Healing System), another raw food pioneer who lived long before Ann Wigmore, said that in order to be healthy, we must eat mucus-less food or a diet that doesn't cause our bodies to make mucus to protect itself. If one eats a diet which causes the chemistry of the body to be acid, then the cells of the body will make mucus to protect them. Over a lifetime, this mucus will do many things. It will be a home for viruses, it will continue to multiply as the body gets more and more acid, it will harden in some places and impede circulation. The acid will also cause the body to hold on to water (weight) in order to neutralize.

So what about the acid alkaline balance? According to naturalhealthschoolonline.com, "over acidity which can become a dangerous condition that weakens all body systems, is very common today. It gives rise to an internal environment conducive to disease, as opposed to a pH-balanced environment which allows normal body function necessary for the body to resist disease. A healthy body maintains adequate alkaline reserves to meet emergency demands. When excess acids must be neutralized, our alkaline reserves are depleted leaving the body in a weak-ened condition."

To adequately understand the acid alkaline balance and the fluids that bathe the cells of the body, think about the experiment performed in the 1930s by Dr. Alexis Carrel, a two-time Nobel Prize winning scientist who performed the first kidney transplant, and was head of the Rockefeller Research Institute. Under his direction a small piece of heart tissue from an embryonic chicken was cultured in a flask. It was provided with nutrients, oxygen and water. The piece of chicken heart was kept growing for more than thirty years, far past the life span of a normal chicken. After thirty-four years, it showed no signs of deterioration. So, the caretakers stopped caring for it and let it die. Carrel concluded that our cells could live and reproduce forever provided proper conditions are maintained.

Dr. Carrel wrote about the experiment in 1935, "When the composition of the [fluid around the cells] is maintained constant [with oxygen, nutrients, etc.], the cell colonies remain indefinitely in the same state of activity. They never grow old. Colonies obtained from a heart fragment removed in January 1912, from a chick embryo, are growing as actively today as 23 years ago. In fact, they are immortal." Alexis Carrel, *Man the Unknown*, New York: Halcyon House, 1938, p. 173.

Theodore A. Baroody, N.D., D.C., Ph.D. in his book, *Alkalize or Die*, said, "The countless names of illnesses do not really matter. What does matter is that they all come from the same root cause too much tissue acid waste in the body!"

A healthy pH body range is 6.0 to 7.5. One can purchase inexpensive pH strips at the local pharmacy and test both the saliva and the urine. "When the pH is unbalanced, the condition forces the body to borrow minerals—including calcium, sodium, potassium and magnesium—from the vital organs and bones and to buffer or neutralize the acid and safely remove it from the body. This strain can cause prolonged damage to the body. Mild acidosis can cause such problems as cardiovascular damage, weight gain, obesity, diabetes, bladder and kidney problems, kidney stones, immune deficiency, premature aging, osteoporosis, joint pain, aching muscles, lactic acid buildup, low energy, and chronic fatigue."

"If acid levels are too high, the body will not be able to excrete acid. It must either store the acid in body tissue (autotoxication) or buffer it—by borrowing minerals from organs and bones in order to neutralize acidity." So...what is the solution? One can gradually begin to de-acidify the body and make it more alkaline! It is as simple as changing the diet. Knowing and eliminating the foods that cause the body to be acidic is important: animal foods such as beef, turkey, chicken, shellfish, pork, fish, eggs, butter, milk, ice cream, cheese, and things like chocolate, carbonated drinks, white sugar, white flour, unsprouted nuts such as peanuts, walnuts, pecans, cashews, etc. A complete list can be found in Baroody's book.

It is very important to add the foods that have the elements that cause the body to be alkaline. The elements which cause the body to be alkaline are oxygen, sodium, magnesium, potassium, and calcium. Wheatgrass and barley grass have chlorophyll which enables the body to make more red blood cells, thus carrying more oxygen. Both are extremely high in magnesium, potassium and calcium. Barley grass is exceptionally high in organic sodium. Also one can add fresh fruits, and vegetables in the raw state, sprouted nuts and seeds of all kinds, and the greens such as parsley, spinach and the lettuces.

Once again, the Ann Wigmore diet proves to be healthful for a set of entirely different scientific reasons!

THE MIRACLE OF MINERALS

by KK Fowlkes

The challenge with the soil in which most of our food is grown is that it has been leached of most of its trace mineral content over the years. As modern farming techniques have evolved, most farms fertilize with NPK (Nitrogen, Phosphorous, Potassium), which will cheaply and dramatically increase crop yields. It is not cost effective for farmers to fertilize their crops with other trace minerals like selenium, calcium, copper, zinc and over sixty others that are needed by the human body for optimum health, so of course, they don't. Over the years crops have depleted the soils of these vital trace minerals.

There is a great debate among wheatgrass gurus as to the best way to grow wheatgrass—using the soil method or growing the grass hydroponically. Some say that the wheatgrass berry has enough energy to form the first 7 inches of wheatgrass and that it takes no minerals from the soil to accomplish this. Those who have grown wheatgrass for a long time point out that after ten days of growing a flat of grass, that there is no soil left!! After cutting the grass, the only thing left is a mat of solid roots--there is no soil. This can only mean one thing.

The grass and roots did in effect take up the minerals and the soil in addition. Looking back a millennia, or a long history of the agricultural activities of the earth think about how people have always grown their food. How? In soil of course. It is only in the last fifty years that we have had such things as hydroponic tomatoes, etc. And the jury is still out as to whether or not these hydroponically grown vegetables are any good at all. Growing healthy nutrient-rich wheat and barley grass that contain trace minerals so essential for good health is crucial for people who are trying to improve their health. The way to accomplish this is first begin with an organic compost and then fertilize the soil in which you grow your grass with a good organic trace mineral fertilizer. So we can add wheatgrass or barley grass to our diets as they are among the best sources of vital life substances on the planet, but only when grown in healthy soil.

If we wish to regenerate our bodies, we can reduce consumption of refined foods, eat more raw enzyme-complete foods, and consider that when we ask for our "daily bread" we remember that the material portion of that request is a direct product of the soil, and if the soil dies, we die with it.

Since we know that most soils are deficient, and we want to now grow some of our own foods in our kitchens (i.e. wheatgrass, barley grass, sunflower greens, buckwheat greens) we will want to start out with the healthiest seed (organic), organic compost, and topsoil possible. Important! We can restore the trace minerals to our soil with an ancient product called Azomite™.

VEGAN & VEGETARIAN RECIPES

SPROUTED/FERMENTED WHEAT DRINK

1. Soak 3 ½ cups wheat or barley 8 to 12 hours.

2. Drain, rinse, and put in sprouting bag or container of some kind.

3. Sprout for 36 hours, rinsing twice per day.

4. Put into gallon jar and fill with clear (filtered if possible) water nearly up to the top (leave enough room for expansion).

5. Put screen or paper towel over the top to keep bacteria in the air from falling in.

6. Let this set for 48 hours until it is fermented (Little bubbles will rise from the bottom).

7. It is now a fermented wheat/barley drink. Sometimes it is cloudy. It should taste rather tart.

8. Strain to separate the grain from the liquid. Store the liquid in the refrigerator for up to 3 days. Drink at room temperature.

9. The remaining seed can be reused twice more to make more fermented drink: Soak 36 hours the second time and 24 hours the third time.

SPROUTED WHEAT CEREAL

1. 2 cups sprouted wheat, 4 cups spring or filtered water, ¾ cup raisins, 1 large apple, peeled, cored or, 1 banana peeled and sliced.

2. Soak raisins in one cup of the spring or filtered water for one hour or until soft. Reserve the water used in soaking the raisins. In a blender, blend wheat with fruit, water and raisin soak-water at medium speed for about two minutes. Use warm filtered water if a warm cereal is desired. The sprouted wheat cereal should have a soupy consistency. Sprouted (hulled) buckwheat, sunflower seeds, or sesame seeds may be substituted for the wheat. (All seeds should be soaked at least 6 hours or overnight.)

LUNCH OR DINNER SALAD

Sunflower greens, buckwheat greens, salad lettuces (if desired), topped with alfalfa sprouts, and/or sprouted fenugreek, add a seed-cheese dressing.

SEED CHEEZ AND SEED SAUCE

⅔ cups hulled sunflower seeds

⅔ cup unhulled sesame seeds

purified water, 3 cups fermented wheat or barley drink

Soak sunflower seeds and sesame seeds separately overnight in purified water. In the morning, rinse sunflower seeds in very warm water to remove skins. Rinse sesame seeds. Put sesame seeds and sunflower into blender. Add ½ cup fermented wheat drink and blend for two minutes. Pour mixture into bowl. Cover bowl with a cloth. Secure with rubber band. Place in warm place with good air circulation. Let stand 6 to 8 hours. Remove cloth. Scrape off top oxidized layer and discard. Spoon middle almost cheese layer into seed bag and hang in the refrigerator overnight, with a bowl under it to catch the liquid. By morning it is Seed cheez. Seed cheez sauce (or dressing) can be made by thinning the Seed Cheese to any consistency desired, using fermented wheat drink as the liquid. Season with Brag's aminos. Seed cheez milk can be made by adding 1 heaping teaspoon seed cheese to an 8 ounce glass of fermented wheat drink. Stir well.

VEGGIE KRAUT

1. Grind 2 heads cabbage (organic cabbage if possible) saving juice, red or white. Use 75 percent cabbage, 15 percent carrots, and 10 percent yam. Add 1 tablespoon Real Salt if you can get it, 2 cloves minced garlic, 1 teaspoon ground dill seed.

2. Put the mixture into a large bowl or crock. Cover with the outer cabbage leaves. Place a large plate and a weight on top. Leave it at room temperature for five days (it can be covered with plastic to keep insects out).

3. Remove scum and leaves. Mix so that the juice is evenly distributed. Cover and place in refrigerator. It should keep for weeks when refrigerated. Some of the juice can be poured off and used to marinate mushrooms or vegetables.

Fermented foods are an aid to digestion, are high in the B vitamins, and are full of enzymes. They provide an acid environment in the bowel whereby favorable bacteria can thrive and overcome unfavorable bacteria. Re-establishing beneficial bacteria to the colon is a major part of many health programs.

GREEN SMOOTHIE SOUP

1. 1 peeled apple (or use watermelon plus white rind in the summertime), 1 cup fermented wheat drink or pure water (if using pure water, add juice of ½ lemon), ½ handful of red dulse (red seaweed; for those who are vegan, salt to taste instead), 1 cup of sprouts and greens (sunflower or buckwheat greens can be used).
   Optional: 1 handful of sprouted mung, adzuki, and peas can add protein to the soup.

2. Blend all together lightly. Add ½ avocado. Blend again until smooth. Enjoy!

SEED CHEEZ VEGGIE LOAF

Mix 2 ½ cups of seed cheese with minced broccoli, green or red pepper, minced onions, celery, etc. Form into loaf. Decorate with red bell pepper or variety of sliced garden vegetables.

ALMOND CREME

1. Soak 2 cups almonds 24 hours. Momentarily dip into boiling water (count to 3 only). Rinse through colander in cold water. Peel-squeeze pointed side out.

2. Put small amount at a time into blender. Cover with fermented wheat/barley drink but not too much—as it won't grind into smooth paste.

3. Let it set 3 to 4 hours and then refrigerate or serve immediately. If you refrigerate before setting the setting takes longer. Almond creme lasts one day.

ALMOND MILK

Add fermented wheat drink to 1 to 2 tablespoons almond crème. Lasts 2 or 3 days.

SPROUTED BREAD

1. 4 to 6 cups wheat sprouts (1 day sprouts),1 teaspoon caraway seeds.

2. Run sprouts through either a grinder, a slow turning juicer with the end screw detached, a Omega™ juicer, or blend in a food processor with a little water. The Omega™ juicer makes a fine smooth dough. Be sure to feed the sprouts into the juicer slowly, so that the motor will not overheat. Mix in the caraway seeds.

3. Press the dough into a small, flat, wafer-like loaf. Place it on an oiled cookie sheet or on a dryer rack, and dry it in a dehydrator or in a warm oven set at 105 degrees. The bread will take from 12 to 20 hours to become crisp.

SIMPLY GREEN DRINK

2 stalks celery
4 large spinach leaves
½ cup parsley
1 ounce of wheatgrass juice
¼ cup water

Wash greens, cut up celery and juice. Dilute with water if desired.

CARROT GRASS

3 carrots
¼ cup water, optional
1 ounce of wheatgrass juice

HAWAIIAN WHEATGRASS

2 cups fresh pineapple juice
1 cup orange juice
1 cup papaya juice
1 ounce wheatgrass juice

Blend

WHEATGRASS SMOOTHIE

2 oranges
1 banana
1 lime
1 ounce of wheatgrass juice
12 ice cubes, crushed

Juice orange, lime and wheatgrass, then place all ingredients in a blender on high speed for 30 seconds.

APPLE GRASS

Juice 1-2 apples
Juice ½ Lemon
¼ cup of water (optional)
1 ounce wheatgrass juice

PURE VEGGIE DELIGHT

2 large carrots
3 stalks celery
½ cup parsley
4 large spinach leaves
½ beet root
½ cup alfalfa sprouts

Wash veggies thoroughly and cut to fit juicer.

TROPICAL PASSION GRASS

2 Kiwi
1 guava or papaya
1 cup pineapple
5 strawberries
1 orange
1 ounce wheatgrass juice

Combine all juices and serve slightly chilled.

SWEET GRASS

2 apples
1 orange
1 ounce wheatgrass juice

ALMOND MILK, GINGER, FRESH FRUIT SMOOTHIE:

Almond milk
Ice cubes
Fresh ginger
Pineapple
Blueberries

Using the freshest (organic) ingredients possible, blend the ingredients above in your Vita Mixer or Blender using whatever quantities of each ingredient per your individual taste.

Makes a delicious, nutritious, quick, healthy breakfast or a refreshing pick-me-up any time of day.

Substitute any seasonal or fresh fruit(s) of your choice in the above recipe.

TAHINI SALAD DRESSING:

2 cups of distilled water
½ cup of fresh lemon juice
⅓ cup of brown rice syrup
1 teaspoon ground cumin
1 tablespoon minced garlic
1 cup of sesame tahini
2 tablespoon fresh chopped basil or parsley (optional)

Combine all the above in a blender except the tahini. Blend well. Slowly add tahini. DO NOT add the tahini until all the other is blended.

Use as a salad dressing or put on baked potatoes.

CAULIFLOWER AND PEAS

1 head of cauliflower
10-12 ounce of baby peas
1 ½ cups rice sour cream
1 tb bragg liquid aminos
2 ts. minced garlic
Dash cayenne pepper
2 tablespoon chopped fresh dill

Steam separated cauliflower florettes until tender, 8-10 minutes.

Steam baby peas for 2-3 minutes.

Combine rice sour cream, garlic, Braggs, and cayenne in a sauce pan. Simmer.

Pour hot sauce mixture over cauliflower and peas. Add chopped dill. Mix thoroughly. Serve immediately.

ALMOST RUM BALLS

1 ¼ cups whole almonds
⅔ cup organic medjoul dates (seeds removed)
1 tablespoon carob powder
1 tablespoon vanilla extract
2 tablespoon brown rice syrup
Coconut flakes, carob powder, or crushed nuts to coat

Puree almonds in a food processor. Add remaining ingredients until well blended.

Form small balls 1 inch in diameter. Roll into balls with palms of hands, not your fingers, to make uniformly round.

Coat the balls with carob powder, coconut flakes or crushed nuts and serve. **Yield:** Approximately 2 dozen.

– Mary Colville Griffith
Delray Beach, Florida

SPROUTED MUNG BEAN SALAD

Boil 4-5 potatoes, then cut in pieces
Chop 5-6 Tomatoes in small pieces
5-6 Onions, finely chopped and cut in small pieces
Cilantro bunch finely chopped
Cucumber 1 finely chopped
lemon juice from 1 squeezed lemon
Sea salt to taste
Green Chili 1 finely chopped

Soak mung beans overnight in water, next day drain the water and tie them in a moist cheese cloth and cover, keep this in a warm place for 10-15 hours and you will see the sprouts coming. Sprouting is good when there is adequate moisture and warmth.

Mix all to the sprouts and serve fresh.

This is an excellent food full of amino acids. vitamins enzymes and minerals.

– Dr. Deepika Sharma

MAGIC BULLET™ BLENDER CUP SMOOTHIE

½ half carrot peeled (sometimes I use the whole carrot)
1 medium peach
1 teaspoon seasame seeds
3 or 4 whole almonds
¼ avacado for thickness
1 tsp of maple syrup (if you like)

Put all ingredients into Magic Bullet™ cup, fill with water, blend and enjoy.

– Emily Guarriello

CREAMY CASHEW ORANGE SHERBET

One ice cube tray of fresh squeezed, strained, sweet orange juice (about 1½ cups).

One ice cube tray of freshly made cashew nut milk *(about 1½ cups, see recipe below).

Freeze both trays overnight or until frozen solid. Blend quickly to make ice cream consistency, a little extra cashew nut milk or orange juice can help the blending process. Serve immediately. If you have a Champion Juicer or similar appliance, you can just run alternating cubes through it. Note that you may get 'streaks' of white/orange, but this just improves the looks, quality and taste of the sherbet. Serve in individual sherbet dishes. Add a sprig of mint on top (optional).

*Cashew nut milk:
Only use 'raw' cashew nuts, not salted nor roasted. (Note: the term 'raw' in this case just means the nuts are not roasted after being shelled, as the shelling process takes heat to dissipate the toxin ingredient within the shells.)

½ cup finely ground cashew nuts, can be made from whole or pieces or raw, cashew nut butter (can also substitute raw, blanched almonds, but not as tasty!)

For richer milk, add more ground nuts.

1½ cups pure, cold water (preferably distilled or spring)
1 vanilla bean pod (optional)

Blend cashews to a very fine consistency. Add cold water and blend well. Strain to remove nut granules. Stir vanilla pod in milk to release vanilla flavoring for about a minute. Use immediately or refrigerate until ready to use.

– Georganna McRoy, Deer, Arkansas

REFERENCES

Many, many people have experienced extraordinary success in meeting their health and well being challenges by using grasses, greens, and sprouts as part of a healthy lifestyle.

One of the longest serving living foods educational centers in the world today is Optimum Health, with Centers in San Diego, California, and Austin, Texas. Based on the teachings and techniques of Ann Wigmore and Raychel Solomon, hundreds of thousands of people have experienced the benefits of this system. From one of our newsletter articles, the following is extracted to give an example of challenges people have met using raw and living foods.

At last, Friday, the end of the second week. On Friday mornings Dan Strobar, one of the long-term staffers at OHI, has what they call "Testimonials." Attendees are invited to share their experiences and observations with everyone assembled.

We hear some extraordinary stories. One of the working guests relates how her bout with breast cancer has gone. She tells us that the doctors had given her little hope after a mastectomy and complications resulted in a suppurating scar that wouldn't heal, and progressive lymph node involvement. She says that after five months on the program, all symptoms have cleared, and the last check up with the doctors left them astonished at the results. She says they deny that diet could have anything to do with the recovery, and are mystified but happy for her. Another relates that their blood sugar levels had dropped to the point where they no longer needed medication. Another said that she had lost a total of eighteen pounds while at the Institute and felt ten years younger. This is just a small sample of the experiences shared during the weekly gathering.

The use of living and raw foods is only a part of an overall lifestyle approach to achieving optimum health. Remember, however, that if you are embarking on a new way of living that involves major changes in your lifestyle, be sure to consult your health-care provider.

REFERENCES

"Bela-Carotene: The Amazing Provitamin that Promotes and Protects Your Health," by Dr. Bruce D. Miller, Institute for Preventive Health Care, Fort Worth, TX, 1985. The vital functions that provitamin A performs in the body. Why you need it in your diet for disease-prevention.

"Clinical Ecology: A New Medical Approach to Environmental Illness," by Iris R. Bell, M.D., Ph.D., Common Knowledge Press, Bolinas, CA, 1982. Geared to physicians. Check it out of your local library and give if to your doctor if you suspect you may be chemically-allergic. Delineates symptoms, introduces concept of toxic body loading.

"Diet for a New America," by John Robbins, Stillpoint Publishing, Walpole, INK, 1987. Stinging indictment of the pesticide industry and use of hormones in meat production, causing premature puberty in children. Presents the need for diet change to nontoxic, whole, live, raw foods.

"Fighting Radiation with Foods, Herbs and Vitamins," by Steven R. Schecter, N.D., East West Health Books, Brookline, MA, 1988. "Documented natural remedies that protect you from radiation, X-rays, and chemical pollutants." Very comprehensive, in-depth coverage of dietary and supplemental health needs for preventing toxic build-up.

"Food Irradiation Facts," by National Coalition to Stop Food Irradiation, San Francisco, 1989. Factsheet explaining why food irradiation is an additional—and needless— threat to our health. Do we want to be guinea pigs for this creator of free radicals in food?

"Food Irradiation: Contaminating Our Food," by Richard Piccioni, The Ecologist, Vol. 18, No 2, 1988. The dangers that food irradiation presents to human health.

"Free Radicals, Stress, and Antioxidant Enzymes," by Zane Baranowski, Biotec Foods, city and date unknown. Explains need for toxin-clearing antioxidant enzymes derived from dried organic wheat sprouts.

"Human Ecology and Susceptibility to the Chemical Environment," by Theron G. Randolph, M.D., Charles C. Thomas, Springfield, IL, 1982. Geared to physicians and pharmacists. Warns about dangerous interactions of toxic chemicals with synthetic chemical pharmaceuticals and synthetic chemical vitamins inside the human body. Why more chemicals, even supposedly therapeutic ones, increase toxic build-up and immune system decline. Why chemical allergy is a warning sign.

"Morbidity and Mortality Reduction by Supplemental Beta-Carotene in CBA Mice Given Total Body Radiation, by Dr.

Eli Seifter, et.al., Journal of the National Cancer Society, November, 1984. Technical paper showing radiation-protection properties of provitamin A in the form of beta-carotene.

"Nontoxic and Natural.- How to Avoid Dangerous Every-day Products and Buy or Make Safe Ones," by Debra Lynn Dadd, J.P. Tarcher, Los Angeles, 1984. If you want to avoid toxic chemicals without altering your lifestyle, this book is indispensable.

"Our Bodies are Dumping Grounds for Toxic Chemicals," by Debra Lynn Dadd, Earthwise Consumer, Mill Valley, CA, Winter, 1989. If you read her book you may want to subscribe to her newsletter. This article reports on latest human adipose tissue survey (conducted annually by the U.S. Public Health Service since 1967). One interesting tidbit: all persons tested showed various levels of styrene in their body fat (styrene is used in fast-food containers [polystyrene]—especially plastic coffee cups).

"The Antioxidants: The Nutrients that Guard the Body Against Cancer Heart Disease, Arthritis and Allergies - And Even Slow the Aging Process," by Richard H. Passwater, Ph.D., Keats Publishing Inc, New Canaan, cr, 1985. Explains how antioxidants neutralize and eliminate free radicals.

"The Art of Making Sprouted Bread," by Steve Meyerowitz, The Sprout House, Great Barrington, MA, 1990. How to do it by the guy who calls himself Sproutman.

"The Beansprout Book," by Gay Courter, Simon and Schuster, New York, NY, 1973. Why sprouts are good for you and good tasting too. Full of recipes and sprouting information.

"The Health Issue of the '90s: Toxic Build-Up," by B.N.G, Inc., Tempe, AZ, 1991. Brochure explains how to stop toxic build-up. Introduces an herbal formula designed to help the body detox itself by drinking Herbal Clean detox tea.

"Troubled Water," by Jonathan King, Rodale Press, Emmaus, PA, 1985. Warns about specific chemical toxin contaminants in drinking water, how they got there and their health effects. Why you may want to get your water tested and/or get a water filtration device.

"Wheatgrass: Nature's Finest Medicine," by Steve Meyerowitz, The Sprout House, Great Barrington, MA, 1990. Why it's good for you and how to make it too.

"Your Home, Your Health and Well-Being," by David Rousseau, W.J. Rea, M.D and Jean Enwright, Ten Speed Press, Berkeley, CA, 1988. Full of how-to suggestions for clearing your home of toxic chemicals and home toxic problems. Includes a chapter by Dr. Rea in layman's terms on toxic body loading. Also discusses chemical allergies experienced by his patients—what is now called ecological illness, confirmed by chemically-revealing blood tests.

NOTES:

NOTES:

NOTES:

NOTES:

WheatgrassKits.com

WHEATGRASS, BARLEYGRASS, SPROUTS, & HERB INFORMATION & GROWING KITS PLUS WHEATGRASS JUICERS

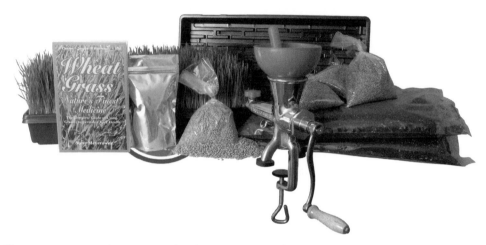

Grow your own wheatgrass, barley grass, sunflower greens, sprouts or herbs for pennies a day! WheatgrassKits.com offers you nature's most perfect living foods.

Find out why over 100,000 people have chosen Wheatgrasskits.com for all their wheatgrass needs. We proudly provide the most complete selection of kits, wheatgrass juicers and supplies to grow wheatgrass, barley grass, herbs, sprouts, greens and edible mushrooms. We also carry soy milk kits, composting supplies, books and more. Check out our information library & wheatgrass blog.

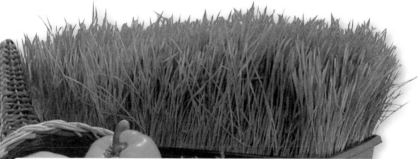

We offer a full line of wheatgrass growing supplies

www.wheatgrasskits.com

COMPLETE & ORGANIC

The Certified Organic Wheatgrass Growing Kit:

- ▷ **5 21" x 10" Growing Trays**
- ▷ **5 bags (5 lbs total) ORGANIC Wheatgrass Seed**
- ▷ **2 Bags Organic Growing Mix-** Forest Based Compost, Completely Animal Free!
- ▷ **Supply of Azomite™**
- ▷ **Wheatgrass, Sprouts, Microgreens and the Living Foods Diet Book**
- ▷ **Growing and Juicing Instructions**

Makes about 50 Liquid Ounces of Juice!

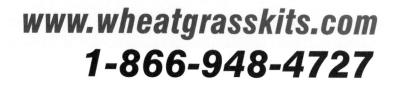

www.wheatgrasskits.com
1-866-948-4727

Handy Pantry Sprouting
Living Whole Foods Inc.

Certified Organic Sprouting Seeds & Sprouting Supplies

Handy Pantry Sprouting has been providing certified organic sprouting seeds and sprout growing supplies for over 20 years now.

Our sprout seeds supplies are perfect if you are new to growing sprouts or a sprouting veteran. Grow Sprouts kits also make a great gift idea!

Find out why tens of thousands of people have chosen Handy Pantry as their exclusive sprouting seeds supplies source to help them grow sprouts with quality:

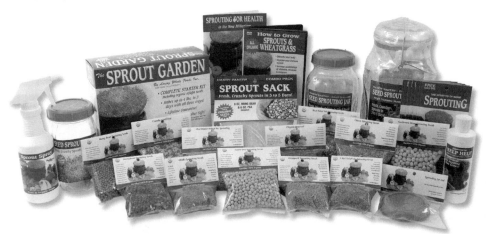

- ▷ **Organic Sprout Growing Seeds**
- ▷ **Sprouting Seeds Assortments**
- ▷ **Sprout Growing Kits**
- ▷ **Sprouters**
- ▷ **Organic Foods and Spices**

- ▷ **Washes & Fertilizers Supplies**
- ▷ **Books & DVDs**
- ▷ **Supplements**
- ▷ **WheatGrass Kits & Juicers**
- ▷ **Food Storage Products**

Growing sprouts on your own is fast, fun, healthy & inexpensive. Just starting in growing sprouts or sprouting seeds supplies and not sure where to start? Start to grow sprouts in no time with one of our Sprouting Seeds Supplies Starter Kits!

www.handypantry.com | www.wheatgrasskits.com

Deluxe Sprout Growing Kit

100% Certified Organic

The Deluxe Sprout Growing Kit:

Provides space saving LIFETIME GUARANTEED stackable sprout kit tray system and a single sprouter lid for soaking the seeds and for making small amounts of sprouts. Everything you need to learn the basic aspects of virtually every kind of organic sprout seed, bean or grain is here for you in this deluxe sprouter pack! A perfect way to get started with sprouts and discover which types of sprouts you like the best. The quantity of seed in these kits makes almost 50 pounds of sprouts!

Kit Includes:

▷ Handy Kitchen Countertop Stackable Sprouter Tray System with 3 Sprouter Trays (Lifetime Warranty).
▷ *Wheatgrass, Sprouts, Microgreens and the Living Food Diet*
▷ 1 Page Sprouter "Quick Reference" Laminated Instructions.

12-Pound Sprouting Seed Assortment - *1 pound each of 12 types of Certified Organic Sprouts Seeds*

▷ 1 Lb. Bean Salad Mix (Adzuki, Lentil, Mung)
▷ 1 Lb. Protein Powerhouse (Garbanzo, Snow Pea, Cabbage, Radish)
▷ 1 Lb. Alfalfa Seed
▷ 1 Lb. Garbanzo (included but not pictured)
▷ 1 Lb. Mung Bean
▷ 1 Lb. Green Clover Seed
▷ 1 Lb. Crunchy Lentil Fest
▷ 1 Lb. Green Lentil
▷ 1 Lb. 3-Part Salad Mix
▷ 1 Lb. Green Pea
▷ 1 Lb. 5-Part Salad Mix
▷ 1 Lb. Radish Seed

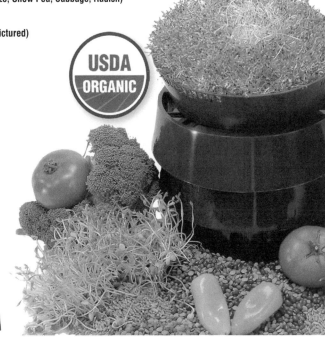

USDA ORGANIC

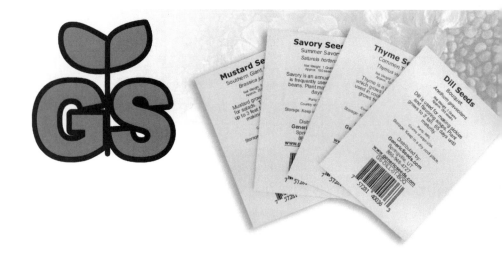

Vegetable seed, Herb seed, Flower seed, and much more!

GenericSeeds.com is your source for seeds for planting, sprouting herbs and vegetable gardening. We carry a wide variety of garden seeds, all at a low price.

All of the seeds at GenericSeeds.com are value priced and inexpensively packaged so we can save you money.

GenericSeeds.com carries all of your vegetable, flower, and herb-garden seed planting needs. Seeds are open pollinated and can be use year after year. If seeds are hybrid it will be specified.

www.genericseeds.com

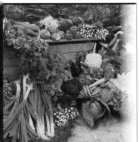
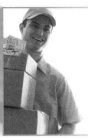
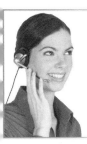

SPROUTING CHART

SEED	METHOD	AMOUNT QT. JAR	SOAK HOURS	TEMP. of	RINSE/ DAY	DAYS	HARVEST INCHES
Alfalfa[1]	Jar/Tray	1½ Tbsp	6 - 8	65-85	2-3x	4 - 6	1½ - 2
Barley	Soil	1-2 Cups	10 - 12	65-85	2x	7 - 10	4 - 8
Bean Salad[1,4]	Jar/Tray	Cup	10 - 12	65-85	2-3x	2 - 5	¼ - 3
Broccoli	Jar/Tray	2 Tbsp	6 - 8	65-85	2-3x	4 - 6	1 – 1½
Buckwheat	Soil	1 Cup	10 - 12	65-80	2-3x	8 - 15	4½ - 6
Chinese Cabbage[1]	Jar/Tray	2 Tbsp	6 - 8	65-85	2-3x	3 - 5	1 – 1½
Fenugreek[3]	Jar/Soil	¼ Cup	8 - 12	65-85	2x	3 - 6	1 - 2
Garbanzo	Jar/Tray	1 Cup	12	65-85	2--3x	2 - 3	½ - 1
Green Pea	Jar/Tray	1 Cup	12	65-85	2-3x	2 - 3	½
Lentil	Jar/Tray	¾ Cup	8 - 12	60-85	2-3x	2 - 4	¼ - 1
Mung Bean[2]	Jar/Tray	Cup	12 - 18	70-85	3-4x	3 - 5	1 - 3
Radish[1]	Jar/Soi1	2 Tbsp	6 - 8	65-85	2-3x	4 - 5	1 - 2
Red Clover[1]	Jar/Tray	2 Tbsp	6 - 8	65-85	2-3x	4 - 6	1½ - 2
Red Winter Wheat	Tray/Soil	1 Cup	10 - 12	55-75	2x	2 - 3	¼ - ½ (grass 6-8)
Soybean	Jar/Tray	½ Cup	12	65-85	2-3x	2 - 5	½
Sunflower	Tray/Soil	1 Cup	10 - 14	60-80	2x	2 - 4	3 - 5
3- Part Salad Mix[1,4]	Jar/Tray	1½ Tbsp	6 - 8	65-85	2-3x	2 - 5	1 – 1½
5-Part Salad Mix[1,4]	Jar/Tray	2 Tbsp	6 - 8	65-85	2-3x	2 - 5	¼ - 3

NOTES:

1. Soak less time during the heat of the summer.
2. Green with light during last day to develop chlorophyll.
3. Grow in dark, allow to soak for a minute when rinsing.
4. Will get bitter if allowed to develop green leaves.
5. Cold final rinse extends storage life.